THE
WHOLENESS
HANDBOOK

THE WHOLENESS HANDBOOK

*Care of
Body, Mind, and Spirit
for Optimal Health*

Elaine V. Emeth
and
Janet H. Greenhut, MD

Foreword by Kenneth L. Bakken

CONTINUUM • NEW YORK

1991

The Continuum Publishing Company
370 Lexington Avenue
New York, NY 10017

Printed in the United States of America

Library of Congress Cataloging-in-Publication Data

Emeth, Elaine V.
    The wholeness handbook : care of body, mind, and spirit
for optimal health / Elaine V. Emeth and Janet H. Greenhut.
        p. cm.
    Includes bibliographical references and index.
    ISBN 0-8264-0519-3 (pbk.)
    1. Holistic medicine.   I. Greenhut, Janet H.   II. Title.
R733.E44 1991
613—dc20   90-44517
                                                          CIP

This book is printed on acid-free recycled paper.

To the One
Who wrote this book in me
and rewrote my life in the process.

—E. V. E.

To the members of St. Luke Health Ministries
for challenging me to grow by your faith, love,
and healing presence.

—J. H. G.

Contents

Foreword

We stand at the dawn of a new era; one that virtually requires us to enter into a process of healing: for ourselves, our families and communities, the world and the earth itself. The technologies of modern life have failed to address the chronic diseases, physical, mental and spiritual, of postindustrialized society. Many of these are in part the result of the destruction and pollution of the biosphere. We systematically rape and plunder our earth. We cling to the "gods of metal" for our defense, rather than the God of our forefathers and foremothers. We push the limits of technology and competition, rather than espouse the hopes of true community and cooperation. We choose death rather than life; brokenness and woundedness over healing and health; fast foods, fast-lane life, and fast religion over fasting, rhythm of life, and authentic spirituality. Then it is no wonder that our world, our institutions, our very lives are being systematically eaten away and undermined. We have forgotten our roots.

Refreshing voices of men and women in medicine, physics, public health, ecology, education, the social sciences, and religious institutions are calling for a public health revolution and a drastic shift in worldview. The time has come to confront the personal and societal structures that trap us in a downward disease-oriented spiral. We are called to break away from our idolatry and addictions (security, affluence, technology, control, power, to name a few) to a radical dependence upon the grace of God.

This is not to advocate an antiscientific bias. Science, in fact, affirms the profound interconnectedness of the cosmos through Einsteinian physics and it verifies the delicate balance of the mind-body relationship through the new field of psychoneuroimmunology. Modern science, therefore, is the foundation for an ecological, whole-person systems approach to health, healing, and health care. Unfortunately, religious institutions have been seduced by a mechanistic, materi-

11

alistic worldview that is outdated, and spiritual life is all too often reduced to a proposition of logic. Modern science is leading us back to the Holy.

The authors of this book challenge the philosophical and theological underpinnings of a dying worldview. This is not a question of *either* rational science and technology, with their limitations and strengths, *or* the nonrational issues of love, faith, hope, forgiveness, and healing. But it is rather a *both/and* proposition. Blaise Pascal states it beautifully, "The heart has reasons that the mind knows not of; do you love by reason?"

St. Paul writes, "Work out your salvation with fear and trembling." "Salvus" is the root word of *salvation*, meaning to be healed or made whole. In order to know graced wholeness and to be fully connected to the life given by God as gift, a person must embrace opposites, must walk through fire and through deep water (Isa. 43:2). Suffering and pain, as well as God's shalom, are very much part of a person's life journey and the life cycle in all of creation. The journey toward wholeness requires truthfulness and courage. Only as we grow and are transformed and integrated, can we enter into solidarity with others. The journey toward wholeness is a path that is often dark and lonely; paradoxically, it is the path to compassion and community.

The authors, Elaine Emeth and Janet Greenhut, are longtime friends and colleagues. Together we have shared the journey—not only in our own personal struggles and joys, but in facilitating transformation and healing for many others. These are women of integrity, who write from the solid grounding of their life experience and professional training. They are women of faith, who witness to the healing presence of YHVH in our world today.

The Wholeness Handbook: Care of Body, Mind, and Spirit for Optimal Health belongs in every home and in the libraries of our educational, religious, and health care institutions. Deeply inspiring, forthrightly informative and practical, this book is rooted in biblical wisdom and sets forth scientific truth, the balance necessary for an authentic journey toward health, healing, and wholeness. There comes a time to speak and to live prophetically within this culture. The time is now.

Kenneth L. Bakken
Seattle, Washington

Introduction

We can experience the optimal health, inner peace, and freedom available to us—even if we happen to have an illness.

We can dramatically reduce the risk of major preventable diseases through changes in life-style and approach to life.

We can avoid creating unnecessary suffering.

We can learn how to care for ourselves and each other in health-promoting, life-giving ways.

How? A paradigm shift, that is, a change in our belief system, or worldview, opens up a whole new realm of possibilities for us. A paradigm is a conceptual framework through which we look at and interpret our experience. This book presents *an overview of health promotion and disease prevention*, looking at this broad subject through a new conceptual framework, which the authors call the wholeness paradigm. This paradigm has six distinctive facets:

1. *The wholeness paradigm is integrated, not dualistic.* Rather than believing that body and spirit are separate (dualism), we look at the human person as an integrated, inseparable whole. Health means wholeness: it must address the physical, emotional, spiritual, and social dimensions of personhood.

Within the current medical model, strictly biomedical answers to the cause of illness have led to impersonal, sometimes aggressive treatments that can do violence to the human spirit. Exclusively psychological or spiritual answers have led to devaluation of our bodies, and untold anguish over such gross oversimplifications as "lack of faith," or casual moral judgments. Inadequate answers often contribute to an increase in suffering, or a substitution of one form of pain for another, rather than truly relieving it.

2. *The wholeness paradigm keeps God at the center.* If we want to see the larger picture, we have to expand the depth and breadth of our

13

vision, setting our sights beyond known horizons, to the point where all disciplines of knowledge meet in One. If we can step back and look beyond our parts, our dimensions, even our individuality, and look *toward* the Wholeness—which is beyond our vision—we can overcome our cosmic nearsightedness. The Wholeness, the Holy— the universal integrity, the integration of the universe—this is the ultimate Mystery we call God. Everyone and everything can be arranged in proper perspective with God at the center.

The current medical model is disease-centered—either having it, treating it, preventing it, or researching it. Often the personhood of the patient and the health-care provider becomes obscured, creating fragmentation, alienation, and limits on what each can give and receive from the other.

3. *The wholeness paradigm is based on a systems approach to understanding sickness and health.* No person gets sick or well in a vacuum. Sickness and health occur within a dynamic context, within networks of relationships, where all people, all nations, and even the planet herself are interconnected. The causes of illness are multiple and complex, and the illness in turn has an impact on the social network around it. The path to healing is unique to each individual. Medicine, psychology, and spirituality each has its respective place, each having valuable contributions to make to the healing process. The wholeness paradigm is *macro*scopic, always looking for the whole picture (which includes the cellular and chemical levels), even though it means giving up simple solutions.

The current medical model tends to monopolize the care of parts of the person: medicine for the body, psychology for the mind, ministry for the spirit, and specializations within each. It prefers to identify a single cause of illness, seeking answers at *micro*scopic levels. It does not deny that the person interacts with the natural, social, and cultural environment, but it finds that parts are more understandable and manageable than the totality.

4. *The wholeness paradigm respects all major faith traditions.* Although the authors' contribution to understanding sickness and health emerges from an identified Christian healing ministry, our perspective is an inclusive one. We want to meet people where they are, without judgment, offering unconditional compassionate presence to all persons, regardless of faith tradition, race, sexual orientation, gender, economics, or any other division. Our intent is always to offer our readers the opportunity to respond to the movement of God within them, within their own faith traditions and their own circumstances.

Also, the authors believe that God is present and active in human lives. Rather than go into a lengthy attempt to "prove" this assumption, we ask our readers who are unconvinced of this assumption to accompany us through our sharing of experience and our way of describing it, and to come to their own conclusions and naming of experience for themselves.

The current medical model places its faith in science, discounting the roles of intuition and the spiritual dimension of life. What is measurable, testable, and replicable is real; everything else is suspect. Those who do believe in nonphysical and nonrational realities find no place for it within the medical model and must integrate those beliefs within their own minds.

5. *The wholeness paradigm avoids sexism.* We attempt to use inclusive language throughout this book. Quotations have been edited for inclusive language whenever possible without creating awkwardness or changing the meaning. Wherever gender-specific pronouns are used in our writing or in quotations, they are meant to be understood as both masculine and feminine. We especially try to use nonsexist language and imagery in reference to God, based on the conviction that persons can never be whole unless we allow God to be whole.

The current medical model is no more and no less sexist than the rest of our culture.

6. *The wholeness paradigm is creation-centered and ecological.* Science in the twentieth century has led us into a realm of possibilities where science alone becomes inadequate. Atomic particles, once thought to be "the building blocks of the universe," are now known to be mostly energy, and highly responsive to other fields of energy and matter. All creation is in motion, interacting with every other part. Physicists are discovering that there are no solids, and nothing is as it appears to be: there are only behaviors, verbs, relationships, and interactions. This leads us to two astounding conclusions: first, that the universe is in the process of being created all the time and we are cocreators in that process; and second, that the origin and the destination of science is rooted in mystery.

The current medical model limits awareness of and involvement with family, work, economic, political, and natural environments. The focus stays on the patient and the treatment of that person's specific disease.

The wholeness paradigm represents a radical departure from the current medical model. The implications for health promotion, disease prevention, and health care provision are far-reaching. These will be explored throughout this book as we apply the wholeness paradigm toward a new understanding of sickness and health, the experience of illness, self-care, social networks, and caring for one another.

The insights we share are informed by experience. St. Luke Health Ministries in Baltimore, Maryland, has provided the context for developing and applying the integrated approach to health care that is offered in this book. From its founding in 1982 by Dr. Kenneth Bakken, until December 1988, St. Luke Health Center in Baltimore has offered the care of physicians, a nutritionist, massage therapists, counselors, spiritual directors, and other supportive and complementary service providers, who worked as a team to treat the whole person in an integrated manner. Within our case conferences, given the diversity of personal and professional skills among the staff, a picture of the whole person would emerge. The people who came to St. Luke Health Center for their health care were presented suggestions and options for their care. They were empowered to become actively responsible for their own health care; in fact, they were called health-care *participants*, rather than clients or patients. This work is being continued at St. Luke Medical Center for pain and stress management in Bellevue, Washington.

The staff and health-care participants who have shared their healing journeys with us have inspired us with their courage, their faithfulness, their joys and their struggles. Again and again, we have seen "more than we can ask or imagine" (Eph. 3:20) be accomplished in people's lives. It is our own stories of healing and their stories that we share to illustrate how persons can respond creatively to life, in sickness and in health. The details have been changed to protect confidentiality while preserving the spirit of our encounters.

Whenever we witness healing, we are confronted with the Holy. Rational explanations fail to provide answers for why some people suffer, why some are cured, why others decline even with the best possible care. When healing occurs, we experience awe, born out of the realization that we can cooperate with healing, but it is not solely our doing. This Mystery, which we name God, is present throughout the journey toward wholeness, and is its destination. We can experience the Holy in the self-preserving ways we survive life's hurts, and in the eventual distress that leads us to change when we are ready. The ability to change, the caring we give and receive, and the abundant new life that results from true healing all reveal God to us.

An appreciation of Mystery in the process of sickness and health does not in any way excuse individuals from responsibility for their own health. As cocreators, we are active participants in healing. God is not Someone "out there" somewhere apart from ourselves—God is present within each person, among us, around us. It is our task to be in touch with the divine spark within us, in other persons, in nature, in technology, and in the humanities. When we are in touch with the Holy, we naturally respond with caretaking that springs from reverence.

This book is written for persons who seek to improve their own physical, emotional, and spiritual well-being, and the well-being of those persons they love and serve. It is for those who are committed to being faithful to their deepest, truest Selves, to God, and to others. The authors assume that the readers include many informed lay persons as well as dedicated professionals. In these pages, we explore the meeting ground of psychology, medicine, and spirituality without using technical jargon: the point here is to communicate and to empower the reader, not to baffle or to create unnecessary dependence on specialists.

The authors sometimes use the unpronounceable Name above all other names, YHVH, out of reverence for the unlimited, unknowable God. YHVH is vocalized as Adonai, the ineffable Name of God, or is respectfully referred to as Hashem, meaning "The Name."

Just as each reader brings his or her own background into the reading of this book, each author contributes unique gifts and perspective.

Elaine Emeth is a Catholic laywoman, whose commitment to healing has led her into a ministry of spiritual guidance, healing prayer, and leading workshops and retreats. She is a graduate of the Shalem Institute Spiritual Guidance Program, and she served as a spiritual director on the staff of St. Luke Health Center for two years. Her educational process has included learning from such teachers and healers as Morton Kelsey, John Sanford, and Sam Keen; the healing teams at the Washington Episcopal Cathedral, Foundry United Methodist Church, and St. Luke Health Ministries; and countless individuals on a quest to heal and to be healed.

Janet Greenhut is a physician and specialist in preventive medicine. She received her MD from Wayne State University, where she also completed her internship. After practicing in a small town in South Carolina with the US Public Health Service, she received her master's degree in Public Health and completed a residency in preventive medicine at Johns Hopkins University. She then served as health center coordinator and staff physician at St. Luke Health Center for two and a half years, where she found her commitment to Judaism was strengthened by her work in whole-person health care. Her current interests are in clinical preventive medicine and work site health promotion.

The authors gratefully acknowledge the staff members of St. Luke Health Ministries who contributed to the original envisioning of this project: Kenneth Bakken, Jim Jenkins, Ann Marie Phillips, SUSC, Bernard Kenyon, and Jon Bishop, MD, and all of the other members of the staff and community over the years who shared their lives, dedication, and ministry. Several careful readers generously gave their personal and professional feedback on various aspects of this manuscript: Kenneth Bakken, DO, DrPH, Nona Brown, Joan Conway, PhD, Daniel Ford, MD, Anne Mason, Peggy Myers, Jerry Overton, Natalie Piescik, Timer Powers, and Joanna Vitale. A special thank you to Carol Bauer Shattuck, who skillfully edited major portions of the manuscript. We are also grateful to our editor and publisher at Crossroad/Continuum, Michael Leach, who believed in *The Wholeness Handbook* from the beginning.

Our families have been loving, supportive, and patient throughout the long months of writing; our deep gratitude to Dan McCarthy; Ilan Gittlen; Tom, Laura, and Margaret McCarthy; Ariela and Nathaniel Gittlen. The faith communities that have nurtured and sustained us include the Community of St. John the Baptist, Foundry United Methodist Church, and Kirkridge. There are no adequate words to thank the midwives to the transformational process of flesh becoming word: a smile, reverent silence, and a prayer of thanksgiving for John Becker, Quinn Conners, Edward Bauman, Dorothy Gentry Kearney, Kasey Kaseman, Charlotte Rogers, and Reed Morrison, who provided companionship and guidance on the inner way.

Authors' Note

Unless otherwise indicated, all biblical references are from the Jerusalem Bible, copyright 1966, 1967, and 1968 by Darton, Longman and Todd, Ltd. and Doubleday and Company, Inc.

The identities of the people written about in the Case Studies of this book have been carefully disguised in accordance with professional standards of confidentiality and in keeping with their rights to privileged communication with the authors.

Part 1

Body, Mind, and Spirit

1

Choose Life!

Y ou are wonderful.

And you are certainly worth taking care of.

On our quest for health, wholeness, and holiness, we can assume that we are remarkable creatures, reflecting the handiwork of our Creator, just as any work of art reveals the spirit of the artist. The spirit that our Creator shares with us is love. As creation-centered theologian Matthew Fox points out, before "original sin," there was original blessing: we are truly, wonderfully made. The true Self is love.

WHAT'S RIGHT WITH YOU?

Life with all of its limitations teaches us from an early age that we are not unconditionally lovable, nor is it safe for us to be unconditional lovers.[1] The love that we are must be hidden in order to survive. The true Self becomes lost to our conscious minds, and it is overlaid with illusions, fears, needs, coping mechanisms, and scars of personal experience.

The true "Self," written with the capital "S," refers to the person we have been created to be. The true Self is both uniquely individual in expression and universal in nature. The true Self is the point of connection with all other persons, all of creation, and God. The Self is not conditioned by personal experiences, and it is limitless in potential. It is characterized by nonjudgmental, unconditional love.

The "self" with the small "s" refers to the ego, or the limited way that we think of ourselves which has been shaped by personal experience. The self includes our beliefs about our strengths and weaknesses, our sense of worthiness, limitations, masks, defenses, judgments, illusions, and fears. As we grow in wholeness, the ego-self becomes more and more accurate as limiting beliefs are stripped away. Then the true Self is allowed into our awareness and can be expressed openly in our lives.

The true Self may be lost to our conscious minds, but it is not lost entirely. For, as Jungian analyst and priest, John Sanford, writes:

> the whole person we are meant to become is unknown to us consciously. Nevertheless, our potential wholeness, the goal of our development, lives within us as a dynamic potentiality that profoundly influences the course of our lives.[2]

Disease commonly occurs when the stirring of the true Self within us disturbs our blind, complacent lives. It can create tension or conflict with the patterns of adaptation that we once needed to survive, challenging us to look at life and ourselves anew, and to reconsider our beliefs about the world. The conflict between our true Selves and the limited lives that we are actually living out produces physical, emotional, or spiritual discomfort or disease. This lack of ease is a gracefull communication of the systems in the body, signaling that the physical, mental, and spiritual needs of the person are not being met. Similarly, surgeon Bernie Siegel teaches that illness keeps our attention on living and loving; it redirects our lives, suggesting that we may not be living our own lives, or that we have forgotten who we truly are.[3]

We usually experience disease or distress of some kind when we are ready to grow. This is not the only circumstance when illness occurs, but it is a common one. There is no point in judging ourselves harshly for being the incomplete persons that we are; our mechanisms for self-protection and survival are necessary, and they serve us well for as long as we need them. When we are strong enough and whole enough to get along without some of our protective behavior patterns and beliefs, our true Selves prod us to let go of these defense mechanisms and to move on.

The great psychologist and thinker of the twentieth century, Carl Gustav Jung, offers this provocative thought on the subject of disease in the form of neurosis or illness:

> We should not try to "get rid" of a neurosis, but rather to experience what it means, what it has to teach, what its purpose is. We should

even learn to be thankful for it, otherwise we pass it by and miss the opportunity of getting to know ourselves as we really are. A neurosis is truly removed only when it has removed the false attitude of the ego. We do not cure it—it cures us. A [person] is ill, but the illness is nature's attempt to heal him [or her] . From the illness itself we can learn so much for our recovery, and what the neurotic flings away as absolutely worthless contains the true gold we should never have found elsewhere.[4]

Acceptance of ourselves, incompleteness and all, is crucial. As long as we judge ourselves harshly or refuse to accept our brokenness, we cannot be healed. Acceptance is the beginning of change. Bernie Siegel writes in *Love, Medicine and Miracles*, "The ability to love oneself, combined with the ability to love life, fully accepting that it won't last forever, enables one to improve the quality of life."[5] He identifies exceptional patients as persons who refuse to be victims, who take charge, make changes, and maintain their dignity and self-respect, regardless of the course of their disease. He goes beyond recommending simple self-acceptance, stating emphatically, "an unreserved, positive self-adoration remains the essence of health, the most important asset a patient must gain to become exceptional."[6]

Self-love is evidenced in Self-discipline, Self-care, Self-affirmation, Self-expression, and Self-protection. And if that sounds self-centered or selfish in a narcissistic way, we can be very clear in stating that it is not: people who grow in Self-discovery invariably find that the true Self *is* love, which cannot be withheld. The true Self is a wellspring that overflows into relationship and Self-giving. We need to die to the limitations of the ego-self, so that the true Self may live.

Until we rediscover the truth of who we are, we are fearful creatures—afraid that who we are is bad; afraid that no one could know us and love us (even God); afraid to let others see the truth about our strengths and frailties; and afraid to look deeply at ourselves. This human failure to accept ourselves is an effective barrier to God's love. We can keep ourselves wrapped in a protective layer of believing that we know ourselves better than God does, grasping the conviction that we are not lovable. Yet Scriptures tell us that God exults with joy over us, renewing us with divine love, dancing with shouts of joy for us as on a day of festival.[7] God dancing with joy over us! We need to pray with the psalmist: "It was you who created my inmost self, and put me together in my mother's womb; for all these mysteries I thank you: *for the wonder of myself,* for the wonder of your works."[8] (authors' italics)

* * *

Physical or emotional or spiritual suffering is not automatically a de-generative experience; in fact, it can be a time of profound personal transformation and discovery. Sometimes we have to fall apart in order to fall together.

Illness is often nature's attempt to heal us, individually or collec-tively. It is one language of the unconscious part of ourselves, the part that insists we become the persons we are meant to be. We need to look at illness as opportunity, because it has something to teach us about ourselves, and about our relationship to others and to God. Therefore, illness has meaning: it can be an invitation, sometimes an imperative, to look deeper within oneself, to grow in truth, and to make conscious decisions that lead to greater freedom and authen-ticity.

Illness can also simply be part of life. There are physical, emotional, and spiritual limits to what a person can endure. Organic, environ-mental, interpersonal, genetic, and possibly even random causes of disease can overwhelm the human body, psyche, or spirit. The chal-lenge becomes finding a way to live fully and deeply, no matter what condition we may face.

We are able to respond creatively to any distress in our lives, whether it is a physical disease, emotional problem, relationship problem, or whatever form the distress may take. A creative response, one that is life-enhancing for one's Self and for others, will lead to greater wholeness, regardless of whether or not the disease is cured.

Health, then, is a by-product of becoming aware of and living out the truth of who we have been created to be.[9] We can develop a lovingly self-disciplined and highly pleasurable way of life for our-selves that enhances discovery of the true Self. This positive Self-care will minimize the risk of preventable diseases and maximize the po-tential for healthy, whole, and holy living, even through experiences of illness and other life experiences. The central requirement is that we learn to care lovingly for our whole Selves.

TOWARD A NEW DEFINITION OF HEALTH

Since we are saying that disease, distress, or illness is usually a com-munication from one part of ourselves to another, and that this occurs when a person is ready to grow, it becomes clear that illness or distress of any kind is often a part of the healing process. Old ways of thinking about disease and its relationship to health and wholeness, and old notions of equating healing with curing will not work for us. We need to consider new models of well-being that allow for disease to be potentially either healing or destroying or a combination of both, rather than assuming that disease is *always* a bad thing. Negative assumptions about disease contribute to persons' feeling bad about feeling bad. This is a waste of time and energy that could be used to get well or to grow.

For the sake of clarity in communication, we propose some definitions for terms used in this book:

Body, the whole physical substance of a person that can be perceived by the senses, i.e., seen, heard, touched. The body is also referred to as the biological, or physiological dimension.

Mind, the dimension of personhood that thinks, perceives, wills, remembers. It is often considered the seat of consciousness, intellect, will, and the personal unconscious (which would include forgotten or denied memories, and latent character traits). Mind seems to be both physical, being located in the brain and in every cell of the body, and perhaps nonphysical as well. It roughly corresponds to the Hebrew *ruach*, the God-given principle that gives life and breath to the body, and is the seat of intellectual function, emotions, and attitude of will.[10] Mind is also referred to in this book as the psychological dimension.

Closely related to mind, and also included in the psychological dimension of personhood, is the capacity to feel emotions, which we call *heart*. This distinction between mind (intellect) and heart (emotions) is often useful in distinguishing between rational, intellectual processes and intuitive, feeling processes. We all experience occasional moments when our minds interpret a situation one way and our hearts perceive the same situation differently.

The emotional dimension of personhood also seems both physical and nonphysical. Anyone who has ever experienced the knotted stomach of anxiety, the lump in the throat of sadness, the crushing pain of grief, the irritation of someone's getting under his or her skin, being scared "shitless," or the heartsickness of love knows that emotions have a physical as well as a mental component. The limbic system of the brain, the processing center of emotions, is an integral part of the autonomic nervous system, which regulates involuntary physical responses.

The quality of heart as the seat of emotions corresponds roughly to the old Hebrew *nephesh*, the essence or the soul or life of the person, again, brought to life by the breath of God. Nephesh is the seat of appetites—hunger, thirst, longing, craving—and the seat of emotions and passions—desire, loathing, sorrow, joy, love, hate, and so on. Nephesh is embodied, and in ancient times, it was seen as residing in the blood.[11] Similar also to our use of "heart" is the Hebrew *lev*, or heart, which describes the center of the human person, the locus of comprehension, and also the determining force in one's conscience and character.[12]

Heart is also used in this book to refer to the deep, still point within the individual, where the person encounters and recognizes the Holy. We sometimes call this place Center, where body, mind, and human and divine Spirit meet. One's "higher Self" resides in this quality of heart and functions as deep wisdom and knowledge.

Spirit, the nonphysical essential part of the person; the life principle that we share with all other persons, with God, and all of creation; the dimension of personhood that drives us to create, love, question, contemplate, and transcend.[13] The spirit may be considered the vital connecting link between God, self, and others; it is our common nature. The sense of self that lives in the human spirit is the true Self, the whole and the Holy within us, the place where we are one. Spirit, as used in this book, seems to correspond to the Hebrew *neshamah*, the very breath of God, by which a person becomes a living, inspirited being.[14]

Illness or *distress* refers to any lack of comfort or ease, whether physical, emotional, spiritual, or social, as it is experienced by the individual who is suffering. This includes sickness, disease, injury, mental illness, neurosis, character disorder, imbalance of any kind, relationship problems, addiction to substances or any other form of enslavement (workaholism, perfectionism, materialism, and so on), abuse, Self-denial, tension, restlessness, and so on, from early warning signs to severe cases. Illness also refers to the impact of disease on the person's social network.

Disease is a biomedical term meaning any physical, mental, or emotional clinical sickness, discomfort, or disability that produces a change in biological structure and functioning. The medical practitioner is generally concerned primarily with disease, which is one component of the illness experience. Arthur Kleinman gives a helpful example in his book, *The Illness Narratives*, which makes the distinction between illness and disease clear:

> When chest pain can be reduced to a treatable acute lobar pneumonia [disease], this biological reductionism is an enormous success. When

chest pain is reduced to chronic coronary artery disease for which calcium blockers and nitroglycerine are prescribed, while the patient's fear, the family's frustration, the job conflict, the sexual impotence, and the financial crisis [illness] go undiagnosed and unaddressed, it is a failure.[15]

Wellness or *health* refers to the absence of physical, mental, or emotional disease. Wellness includes optimal functioning of body systems and psychological processes appropriate to one's age. It means internal harmony between organs and body systems, and external harmony as evidenced in the ability to interact with one's natural, social, technological, and spiritual environment.

Health and wellness also refer to conditions that are better than simply "not sick," but are still incomplete and therefore less than the fullness of life that we will call "whole" or "holy." The World Health Organization defines health as "a state of complete physical, mental and social well-being and not merely the absence of disease or infirmity."[16] It also describes health as "the optimal functioning of the human organism to meet biological, psychological, ethical, and spiritual needs."[17]

The Christian Medical Commission describes health as "a dynamic state of well-being of the individual and the society; of physical, mental, spiritual, economic, political and social well-being; of being in harmony with each other, with the natural environment and with God."[18]

Wholeness and *holiness* are used in this book to describe the full realization of the individual in open, dynamic relationship with God, others, and all that is. This wholeness, or holiness, is the goal of the journey, whether we call the process self-actualization, individuation, healing, or whatever name we give it. We can achieve a *degree* of wholeness or holiness, but it is never totally achieved in our lifetime. It is beyond our knowledge, or even our imagination; perhaps it can be described as the perfect living out of complete union with God.

Healing is the process of growth toward wholeness and holiness; *curing* is the process of overcoming a state of disease and becoming healthy, or well. (We return to the relationship between healing and curing.)

It is important to remember that although we must define body, mind, and spirit to be able to write and talk about them, we view them as inseparable: dynamic, interactive, each dimension of the person having a profound impact on every other dimension of personhood. Ashley and O'Rourke write in their work on health-care ethics:

Every human act is an act of the whole person, involving spiritual, ethical, psychological, and biological dimensions. Every human biological function has human (and therefore spiritual and ethical) significance, and conversely even our most spiritual activities involve the body and must respect the structure and functioning of the body.[19]

At St. Luke Health Ministries, we used a "bent-axis model" of well-being that was presented by Kenneth Bakken in *The Call to Wholeness*. This model continued to evolve out of our experience of sharing people's healing journeys.[20] See Figure 1-1.

On the left we see the descending vertical axis, which we describe as "Living in Neutral." This represents a path of disintegration, beginning with simple lack of awareness that leads to early warning signs and symptoms, which may progress to disease, further disintegration, and possibly premature death. The motivating force that propels individuals on this downward path is fear. It is fear of facing the truth, of making changes, of letting go of old patterns and beliefs that makes it seem easier to coast along avoiding issues, than it is to choose abundant life with all of its honesty, freedom, and responsibility. Typically, the fear is not even conscious; living in neutral is often simply being unaware.

The horizontal axis depicts the path of growth toward wholeness and holiness. The motivating force behind the movement toward wholeness is love. Love for God, self, and others leads persons to grow in awareness, which leads to understanding, transformation, greater integration, and wholeness.

Disintegration is an essential component of reintegration and becoming more whole. Change cannot take place without some discomfort. Integration requires that old ways come apart, so that they can be put back together in a new way. The notion of rebirth, new creation, resurrection themes, transformation, all involve dying to illusions or to self, letting go, loss, or other forms of distress, including the possibility of disease or illness. We have to be careful to avoid thinking of disease and wholeness as mutually exclusive. Sometimes disease is a necessary part of a person's journey toward wholeness. Jungian analyst and Episcopal priest, John Sanford, says of the healing, or individuation, process:

Individuation is in itself a kind of wound, and there is a connection between becoming whole and experiencing one's illness and woundedness. We can even speak of individuation as a "divine wound."[21]

FIGURE 1-1.

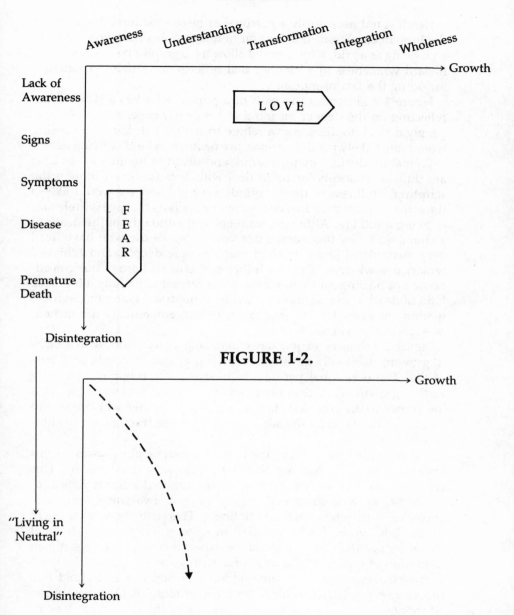

FIGURE 1-2.

Death is not necessarily a personal or medical failure; it is a part of the human condition. It is helpful to imagine this bent-axis model of well-being as a grid, which would allow us to graph a person's journey toward wholeness in a manner that reflects our human experience, including the fact of mortality.

Figure 1-2 illustrates the path of a person who has a habit of not reflecting on the deeper meaning of his or her experience, and who simply drifts into disease as a refuge from life. This life of not seeing would most likely result in premature death, or a kind of living death.

Premature death, "living death," and death in the fullness of time are difficult concepts for us to deal with because, even though the scriptural "fullness of time" sounds very old and we would like to think that is what it means, our experience tells us that age is irrelevant to living a full life. Although we rebel at the thought of the death of a child, we know that sometimes young people die who have lived very meaningful lives, touched many people deeply, and achieved remarkable wisdom. The death that concerns us here in our consideration of healing and wholeness is the refusal to be fully alive. This kind of death is exemplified in "living in neutral," going through the motions of everyday life mechanically and emotionally untouched, or even in the will to die.

Figure 1-3 reflects the journey of a courageous person, who is open to growth, habitually questions everything, and responds with love of life. The occasional periods of disease become opportunities for further growth and a deepening embrace of the fullness of life. This life comes to an end, too, but in a place of greater wholeness and holiness, illustrated by the advancement toward the right on the horizontal axis.

Figure 1-4 similarly shows the path of a courageous person, in this instance, one who has not enjoyed particularly good health. This could be the journey of a person who suffered chronic illness or disability, but who continued to love, grow in awareness, and make choices for life, wholeness, and holiness. This path shows movement to the right on the horizontal axis, in spite of illness. Even death at an earlier age than one's normal life expectancy is not necessarily an indication of a person's having refused to grow.

The challenge for us in this model is to find a way to hold two separate, but related, continua in creative tension. One continuum addresses sickness, disease, and health, and the movement toward health that we speak of as "curing." The other continuum addresses fear and lack of awareness, and love and wholeness, with the movement toward wholeness being called "healing." The two are related,

FIGURE 1-3.

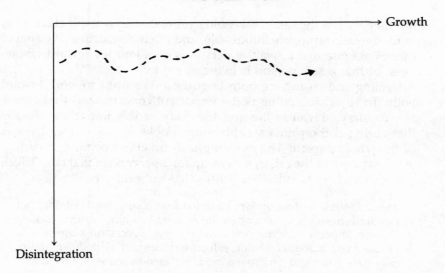

FIGURE 1-4.

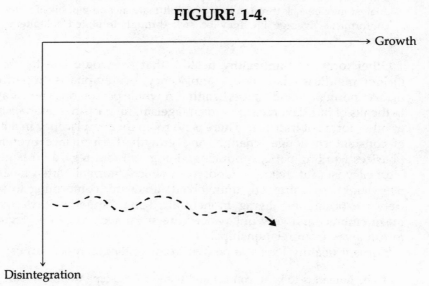

but they are not the same. Sweeping generalizations about either one, or their relationship, are impossible, and often destructive. We simply cannot assume that a healthy person is on a journey toward whole-ness, or that a sick person is living in neutral.

Healing and curing are both important. We want to work toward both. To say that healing is the important concern, and that curing is secondary, devalues life and the body as less important. To say that curing is the primary concern overlooks the dignity and needs of the whole person. The overemphasis on either healing or curing, at the expense of the other, sets us up for a perversion that Paul Tillich calls "unhealthy health." He writes that unhealthy health

> comes about if healing under one dimension is successful but does not take into consideration the other dimensions in which health is lacking or even imperiled by the particular healing. Successful surgery may produce psychological trauma; effective drugs may calm down an un-easy conscience and preserve a moral deficiency; the well-trained ath-letic body may contain a neurotic personality; the healed patient of the analyst may be sick through lack of an ultimate meaning of his life; the conformist's average life may be sick through inhibited self-altera-tion. . . .[22]

Other forms of "unhealthy health" that we would like to avoid include mindless adaptation, complacency, overemphasis on perfor-mance, normalcy, and "superhealth." A whole person does not adapt to the ills of our day: racism, sexism, ageism, militarism, materialism, or other forms of injustice. There is no room for complacency in a life of constant challenge, change, and growth. Performance overem-phasizes working parts, producing, doing, without regard for being. Normalcy is an unreliable standard in which "normal" often means overweight, overstressed, uninvolved, unaware, conforming to so-ciety's expectations, living in neutral. Being "superhealthy" may mean embracing a very unbalanced life-style, such as using jogging to run away from relationships.

Nor is it healthy for us to be free from conflict. Sanford writes:

> To be human is to be in conflict and there is no escape from this. Not everything in the psyche is compatible with everything else. . . . It is almost certain, in fact, that the inner demands of the unconscious will conflict with the demands, expectations, and rules of others around us, and society in general.[23]

Sanford goes on to say that the journey toward wholeness is the way of the cross, requiring that we find a way to carry the burden of our own psyche's opposing tendencies. This is supported by Jesus' exhortation that those who would be his followers must renounce themselves, take up their crosses, and follow him.[24]

Rather than seeking peace, comfortableness, health in one dimension, adaptation, normalcy, or any other imposter for true wholeness, we need to look at life, with all of its dimensions, struggles, conflicts, and rewards, and say "yes" to all of life. Consider the message of Rabbi Harold Schulweis:

> For Judaism life is holy—not life in another time or another place, not life in heaven among angelic forms—but this one here and now with all its human agonies and frustrations. There is basic to Judaism an intense thirst for life.
>
> Life is the major attribute of God—[God] is chai ha-olamim, life of the universe. To desire life is to desire God. To destroy life in oneself or another is to loathe God. We are bidden to fall in love with life again, to seize hold of this day and rejoice in its marvel.[25]

GOD'S PRESENCE AND ACTIVITY IN OUR LIVES

We can name attributes of God, such as Life of the universe, Love, Truth, Justice, Mystery, and Wisdom, but we cannot name or define God. God is infinite, beyond our ability to know or even to imagine. The unpronounceable name, YHVH, respectfully attempts to refrain from reducing God to something manageable for our finite minds to grasp. Our human tendency is to want to make God in our own image, or to fashion a God that is useful to us.

The question of how present and active God is in our lives is answered in highly individual ways, depending on our concept of God and how we name our experiences in life. Some would say that God is extremely active in our lives, even to the point of providing parking spaces, helping on tests, and making sure a favorite team wins in sports competition. Others who experience the same benevolence in life of finding needed parking space, feeling the professor asked the "right" questions (the ones they knew the answers to), and whose favorite team often wins would not think of assigning their happy experiences to God's direct intervention.

Similarly, when people who believe that God is directly involved in life's affairs experience suffering, they will describe that painful experience as a blessing, a chastisement, persecution by the devil, or any other description that fits into their belief system. Still others who suffer, but who believe in God and feel that God is less directly involved, might explain their experience in terms of God having set the universe on course, allowing the free will of humanity, caring intensely about the consequences of our human mistakes, but not intervening—a God who suffers with us.

How can we remain open to the infinite and image-less God, and name our experience of God, without confusing the reality of God with our inadequate attempts to describe our experiences? For, as Thomas Aquinas wrote: "Then alone do we know God truly, when we believe that God is far beyond all that we can possibly think of God."[26]

Our understanding of healing comes from listening to people— people who claim miraculous healings, people with chronic illnesses or handicaps, people who struggle with mental illness, people in health-care professions. Invariably, there comes a point in the conversation, whether the person is "religious" or not, when the person falls into thoughtful silence and out of that silence comes a very quiet conclusion: healing is a mystery. Not just a "mystery," like a riddle we cannot grasp, but Mystery—the work of the Infinite Lover in our lives. There is some power, or Someone, beyond ourselves, that originates outside of our human wills and our limited consciousness, that moves us toward wholeness. This power has traditionally been called grace, and is described as God's own life, or God's love.

We experience the healing, life-giving, creative power of God both within ourselves and surrounding us. The divine nature within us, called the immanence of God, can be manifested in many ways, one of which is the grace that moves us toward wholeness. Other experiences of God's immanence include creativity, empowerment, insight, commitment, and longing for God. God also touches our lives, challenges us, and changes us through sources outside of ourselves; this is called the emanence of God. These sources of contact with the Holy include nature, community, worship, reading, music and the arts, and relationships with other people.

Healing is not so much our quest for God as it is God's quest for us. In our more reflective moments, we know that all of our seeking is but a response to God's initiative. We become more whole and more holy when we respond with love.

RESPONSE-ABILITY

The question of responsibility for disease haunts us. Too often it is a thinly disguised question of who or what is to blame. Throughout history, human beings have wrestled with the problem of suffering, trying to understand why people suffer, and attempting to find meaning in that universal experience. All of our answers have serious shortcomings, and inevitably cause further suffering, which is unnecessary and counterproductive. Whether we perceive illness as a result of forces outside ourselves, such as pollution, cultural stress, germs, heredity, allergy, or weather, or as a result of forces from within ourselves, such as life-style choices (diet, exercise, and so on), karma, the demands of our unconscious, or even God-within, we find ourselves either cast as victims, or burdened with guilt. Our "answers" to the problem of human suffering always have loopholes and inconsistencies, which raise more painful questions: Why do innocent children suffer? Why do plants and animals become sick? Why do some loving, giving people die young? Simple answers are simply inadequate. The fact remains: suffering is. Our task is to respond. Responsibility is just that, response-ability. We are able to respond.

God of laughter and surprise and paradox invites us to discover the blessing in everything, including apparent failures. When we look at the whole of our lives without denial, owning our brokenness as well as our strengths, our difficult emotions as well as our "nice" ones, we meet God in unexpected places: we are astonished to find forgiveness in failure, healing in our woundedness, freedom in truthfulness, new life in barren places, God in our everyday lives. Our illnesses can be full of grace, a catalyst for change that carries us to greater wholeness and authenticity. How, then, can we move beyond states of illness and disease? If disease is part of the healing process, is being free of disease an appropriate goal?

As people of faith, the *only* appropriate goal that holds up in every circumstance is to try to keep God, who is Truth, at the center of our lives. Our goal, then, is to be attuned to the truth, which is to deepen our relationship and harmony with God, self, and others. Our understanding of what this growth in relationship means and what it requires of us is deepened through prayer. Prayer is simply opening ourselves to God, who waits and is available to us. Ken Bakken, founder of St. Luke Health Ministries, wrote: "Living in wholeness is opening ourselves, according to our capacity, to the divine light of God."[27] The divine light reveals to us who we really are. We begin to see ourselves and our world through "God's eyes."

Healing is a by-product of living one's own life, becoming the person he or she is meant to be, learning to live and to love without reservation. Ken Bakken describes the task for a Christian in his book,

The Call to Wholeness: "The central point is to seek *first* the [Reign of God] and then everything else will come in its proper order, including health."[28] Other contemporary writers and healers confirm the necessity of keeping authentic living and loving as our personal goal: Bernie Siegel's work with exceptional cancer patients; Sam Keen's workshops on dis-ease, myth and self-healing; Louise Hay's work with persons with AIDS; Steven Levine's work with persons "healing into life and death"; Jerry Jampolsky's learning from children with terminal illnesses and their families; the staff at St. Luke Health Ministries; and countless others. Healing will follow, *whatever healing means in each individual situation*, regardless of whether one's disease is cured or not.

We may not know how to define healing in a particular case in advance, but the divine spark within us will recognize the healing when we witness it, and it will be holy. Perhaps for one, healing will mean coming to terms with self and experiencing a sense of deep peace as one is dying; for someone else healing may mean a complete physical cure; for another it could mean discovering that she or he is loved through the caretaking received during the illness; for many it involves reconciliation with others, God, or self.

Making the inward journey toward wholeness is not something that anyone else can do for us. The actions that grow out of this inward journey—life-style choices, health habits, commitments, work, loving actions—can only be lived out by the person who has made the inward journey. An adult has ultimate response-ability for his or her own health. Health-care providers have a supportive role. They can perform the valuable service of relieving symptoms, monitoring the process, and/or creating the environment for deep, lasting healing to take place. Ideally, a physician will empower a patient by giving that person the diagnosis, treatment, and information needed to make his or her own choices and changes.

A wide range of creative responses to disease is explored in detail in the course of this book. The question is always, How can I respond with love? The assumption here is that being faithful to yourself, and doing what is loving for yourself, will be best for you and for everyone else around you, and that doing what is loving for others around you will also be best for you. This love cannot be selfish or Self-sacrificing, for neither of these is truly loving. Love has many faces: sometimes it is gentle, sometimes challenging, but it is always free-flowing and life-giving.

Creative, loving response-ability implies that we are not alone. People do not get sick, or well, in a vacuum.

WE ARE ALL IN NEED OF HEALING

We are all pilgrim people on our way toward wholeness and fullness of life. Healing is a process that leads us toward becoming the whole, unique persons whose potential lies within us, but wholeness is never completely achieved in our lifetime. We are always on the way.

Some people appear to be healthy and whole but, in fact, they may simply be more able to conceal their incompleteness, or they may be in more peaceful places on their journey. Perhaps the persons who are farthest from wholeness and the most resistant to growth are the ones who believe that they are no longer "on the way" because they have "arrived."

Any separation between "the sick" and "the well" is simply an illusion that protects those who perceive themselves as whole and well from their vulnerability and incompleteness. This unfortunate illusion also sets us up so that a person who enjoys good health may feel superior, and a person who happens to be sick may feel inferior. Once we eliminate the illusion of separation between sick persons and healthy persons, we realize that we are all incomplete and in need of healing, and compassionate presence to one another becomes possible.

The healing process itself requires disintegration and reintegration as we become aware of the truth of ourselves, step by step, and integrate each new insight or change. Growth is frequently painful, since it requires letting go of illusions, false security, control, and old beliefs in order to make room for new beliefs, understanding, humility, and vulnerability. Disease is often the graced moment when new learning is possible, or new insight breaks through to our awareness.

There is no reason to feel bad about feeling bad. We must learn to be gentle with ourselves and forgive ourselves for being less than whole. Much relief is to be had by putting a stop to some of the ways we commonly add to our own suffering, such as assigning guilt or blame, becoming discouraged with our progress, or making comparisons with other people.

The journey toward wholeness can feel discouraging at times, as we face the same old wounds and personal issues that we thought we had already resolved. Many courageous travelers on the inner way have found that the path toward wholeness is not a straight highway that forges ahead steadily. Rather, it is a spiral path that requires one to go over old issues again and again, but at deeper and deeper levels of insight and healing.

Rather than become bogged down with guilt, blame, discouragement, or comparisons, we need to get on with the work of naming our own present situation truthfully and responding to the present challenge.

Compassion calls for an inner gentleness that is born of true humility. Humility is owning all of our humanity, strengths, and weaknesses, without exaggerating any of these, realizing that everyone has his or her own unique set of strengths and weaknesses. When we try to conceal our weaknesses, or deny or hold onto our "negative" emotions, we become too cluttered to be able to be open to others in a compassionate way; we have set ourselves apart in a pretense of being different, or better, or worse than other people.

Henri Nouwen describes the inner housekeeping that is necessary for compassionate presence in his book, *The Genesee Diary*:

> Today I imagined my inner self as a place crowded with pins and needles. How could I receive anyone in my prayer when there is no real place for them to be free and relaxed? When I am still so full of preoccupations, jealousies, angry feelings, anyone who enters will get hurt. I had a very vivid realization that I must create some free space in my innermost self so that I may indeed invite others to enter and be healed. To pray for others means to offer others a hospitable place where I can really listen to their needs and pains. Compassion, therefore, calls for a self-scrutiny that can lead to inner gentleness.
>
> If I could have a gentle "interiority"—a heart of flesh and not of stone, a room with some spots on which one might walk barefooted—then God and my fellow humans could meet each other there. Then the center of my heart can become the place where God can hear the prayer for my neighbors and embrace them with his love.[29]

Bernie and Bobbie Siegel speak of healers as "privileged listeners." In order for others to feel safe enough to share their pain with us, they need to know that they will not be judged. Those of us who know that we are ALL in need of healing also know that we are all in this process together, and no one is in a position to judge anyone else. When we are trusted as privileged listeners, we cannot help but understand our neighbors, and feel a sense of awe at how gracefully people survive and grow.

Fortunately, as members of families, neighborhoods, and faith communities, we are not all in disintegrated stages of healing or in healing crises at the same time. Those who have experienced some healing in their own lives are able to be living reminders of God's presence to those who are presently in pain, offering empathy and hopeful trust based on a long corporate and personal history of God's faithfulness. We can be privileged witnesses to the wonder of God's grace at work in an individual's life—the grace that carries that person toward wholeness, is his or her comfort and strength through the process, and empowers the person to respond faithfully. Sanford observes: "A certain faith in the healing process is generated by having found healing oneself, not to mention a capacity for empathy with those who are ill, which can only come through having suffered."[30] Since the healing journey seems to be a deepening spiral, we can be sure that those who have known healing will know it again, and again, and again.

Healing is always communal—we must give and receive, share our gifts generously, and receive from others with gratitude. Dr. Stuart Kingma's words express a reality that undergirded our work at St. Luke Health Center: "To be human is to be 'in community,' to see ourselves as neighbors, interdependent, living together, accessible and perhaps even living for the other."[31]

We must move beyond seeing ourselves as isolated persons on individual healing journeys. The human family, indeed, all of creation, pulsates with divine energy. Our choices for life and death, and our sickness and health, have a profound impact on the whole. According to Bakken, "We must begin to ask the questions that will lead to reconciliation and healing, individually and corporately, and ensure the survival of our planet."[32] There are no individual decisions: to choose life for one's self is to choose life for us all.

2

Understanding Illness

THE SEARCH FOR MEANING

Suffering without meaning is intolerable. The universal experience of suffering has been a major motivating force behind the religious quest of humankind. Every religion attempts to wrestle with questions about how and why we suffer. If we can find a way to give meaning to our experience, then suffering becomes more bearable.

Primitive societies seem to have an advantage with regard to giving meaning to the experience of suffering. They attend to illness within a social, spiritual, and environmental context. Studies of shamanic healing across cultures, continents, and history show amazing similarities. One predominant characteristic of shamanic healing in primitive groups is that healing practices are tightly interwoven in a system of shared beliefs. Their corporate religion seeks harmony with the natural world and the unseen, spiritual dimensions of life. Among primitive peoples disease is generally viewed as an intrusion from outside the person, such as an evil spirit, an arrow, or some other invasive element, but the main concern is what caused the afflicted person to lose his or her power of self-protection. Bodily ailments are seen as moral, spiritual problems that cause a disruption in the open communication between the person and his or her world. Trance, rituals, community involvement, and medicinal plants are used by a shaman, who is the equivalent of a combination of our modern physician and priest, to restore power, balance, and harmony to the diseased member of the tribe. The goal of the society and the goal of healing are the same: spiritual development as evidenced in a dynamic, harmonious relationship with the cosmos.

Similarly, every health system reflects societal beliefs as to the purpose and meaning of life, whether these beliefs are articulated or not. One might infer from modern health-care delivery systems in America today that ours is a corporate religion that emphasizes keeping people productive, affirms the primacy of technology, denies death, finds suffering unacceptable, medicalizes life transitions, and maintains the separation of mind, body, and spirit as the specialized domains of psychologist, physician, and priest.

And yet many health-care providers are frustrated by the boundaries of their specializations, the limitations on their time with their patients, the adversarial climate created by the threat of malpractice suits, the inequities in provision for the poor and uninsured, and other conflicts with their commitment to healing. Even though the usual system supports depersonalization and fragmentation, wisdom, compassion and justice are often found in certain individuals within the system. These genuinely wholistic health-care providers resonate deeply with Sir William Osler, a Canadian physician who practiced during the late nineteenth and early twentieth centuries, who said that it is more important to know the patient who has the disease than the disease the patient has.

One such voice out of the wilderness of impersonal health care is that of Arthur Kleinman, MD, author of *The Illness Narratives*. Kleinman makes the distinction between disease and illness: disease meaning the change in biological structure or functioning that is the concern of the health-care practitioner; illness meaning the lived experience of the sick person and his or her social network as he or she perceives the condition, lives with it, and responds to it. Illness refers to the human experience of suffering and how it fits into the individual's whole life, as well as the lives of the persons close to him or her. Consequently, two different healing functions are called for: controlling the disease, and attending the process of finding meaning in the illness.[1]

Both healing functions must be provided in order for true healing to take place. Some physicians may be well suited to offer both functions simultaneously; in other cases, a collaboration of persons with differing gifts can meet the needs of the person who is ill. The interdisciplinary team approach has worked well for the staff and participants at St. Luke Health Center. Here participants have been relieved of the endless trek from doctor to psychologist to minister to social worker to physical therapist in a quest to get their needs met.

The wholeness paradigm developed at St. Luke Health Center is a worldview that seeks to keep God at the center, and sees each individual as an open system in dialogue with all of life, including other persons, the natural world, and the divine. The goal of health care is to enable the participant to enter more fully into an authentic relationship with God, self, others, and creation. The immense practicality of the wholeness paradigm will become more clear as we turn now to focus on a systems approach to understanding illness, and then to explore some of the common levels of illness experience that we have frequently encountered in our practice.

A SYSTEMS APPROACH TO ILLNESS

Generally speaking, medical research has been oriented toward identifying a single cause, or "specific etiology," of illness in order to treat the disease and/or to prevent it. This type of research, which is based on the belief that every disease is caused by a specific identifiable microorganism, has led to one stunning scientific discovery after another. In the last century, several major illnesses have been virtually eradicated or brought under control. Vaccines have been developed for rabies, tuberculosis, and polio; insulin was isolated and made available to treat diabetes; sulfa drugs, penicillin, and other antibiotics made other potentially fatal illnesses treatable. Medicine has also made tremendous strides in surgery, organ transplants, diagnostic tools, anesthesia, and many other areas.

There is a growing recognition of several "nonspecific" elements of medical practice as well. These include such factors as doctor-patient relationship, hopefulness or helplessness, touch, the patient's support system, and the belief system of both doctor and patient. These nonspecific elements are much more difficult to research and evaluate because the nonspecifics are, by definition, difficult to isolate.

Although researchers are able to establish that particular psychological, social, genetic, environmental, or spiritual factors have an impact on illness, it is difficult to translate these findings into a program for health promotion and maintenance. Part of the problem is that it is one thing to say, for example, that hope is crucial to a person's ability to get well, but no one can say truthfully that hope alone will cure in all cases, or that being hopeful will prevent disease.

The reality is that illness and disease are very complex. There are multiple causes, each of which is interacting with every other factor. The doctrine of specific etiology identifies the single *essential* cause of a disease: for example, one cannot have strep throat without the presence of the streptococcal bacteria. But a systems approach is required to explain why a person becomes ill at a particular time, or how the same person is able to resist infection in the presence of the same bacteria at another time.

The systems approach is a radically different way of thinking compared to the usual linear, cause-and-effect, or even multiple-cause thinking. Traditionally, in a linear chain reaction, we are trained to watch for A to cause B, B to cause C, and so on. In a multiple-causation model, we would envision A, B, C, and D to each have an impact on E. The systems model, in contrast, is characterized by the presence of many factors, each of which has an impact on every other factor. It is very dynamic, and comes closest to describing our experience of illness.[2]

Using the systems model, we recognize that a host of factors, such as microorganisms, genetics, health habits, family, society, environment, beliefs, stress, and personal meaning all have a role to play in the experience of health and illness, and that all of these factors have an impact on each other. It is important to remember that affirming the importance of one element of the disease process does not negate the significance of any other element. Any or all of these factors may be present in various combinations in each individual's circumstances. Research affirms the interconnections, but is unlikely to come up with a simple formula—there are simply too many variables.

How does systems theory apply to real-life illnesses?

Suppose a healthy respiratory therapist comes down with pneumonia. It does not seem surprising, considering all the sick people he treats in the hospital. He is exposed to many different kinds of bacteria every working day. He goes to see his doctor, who diagnoses the illness, prescribes an antibiotic, and sends him home to rest.

Most medical problems we have begin and end this way. The physician looks for the specific cause of the symptoms and then, if possible, treats that illness. When the symptoms and signs of the illness resolve, then the patient is cured. However, it does seem strange that a healthy person who is exposed all the time to the same bacteria should fall ill at one particular time and not at another. If we look beyond what agent caused the illness, then we may find ourselves asking: Why did *this* person get sick? And why now?

For instance, we may find out that the respiratory therapy department has laid off a number of people and this therapist has had to work one or two double shifts per week. His wife had a baby four months ago and she is tired and irritable. She cannot understand why he has to work so much when she needs him at home. The addition of a family member has put a financial strain on the family, especially since the therapist's wife is no longer working outside the home. He is always aware of the threat that he may be the next one laid off in his department.

Most of us would have no problem recognizing that this man is "under stress." Our own experience tells us that when we are in a comparable situation we are more susceptible to illness. Many factors influence our state of health; the agent of the disease is only one of them.

The biomedical model tells us that disease occurs when there is a derangement at the cellular or molecular level. Pneumonia occurs when certain lung cells become infected with a bacterium. A person gets cancer when one cell starts to divide uncontrollably and evades the immune system.

In this predominantly linear model, disease is seen as originating with the "agent" (bacteria, cancer cell). Treatment logically then is aimed at eliminating or at least controlling the agent of disease. In these cases, the patient with pneumonia would be given an antibiotic, and the one with cancer might be treated with chemotherapy or radiation.

The systems model of disease causation, in contrast, puts the individual not at the top of a hierarchy of systems but in the middle. Here we see that people are affected not only by what happens within their own bodies but also by the social and biological systems outside themselves. See Figure 2-2.

Communication in this hierarchy does not just occur in a linear fashion, as from Community to Family to Person. We get information from all parts of the hierarchy. As soon as we go outside, for example, we know what the weather is. The information does not have to be sifted down from Biosphere to Person through the intermediate levels.

With this systems model, disease is seen not as the simple result of an invasion of the body by a foreign substance or of an uncontrolled growth of a cell. Instead, we become aware that disease is the consequence of a constellation of circumstances. Looking back at the respiratory therapist, for example, we can see that the disturbances in his family and job may have contributed to his susceptibility to illness. Therefore, bacteria to which he was normally resistant were able to invade his cells and cause pneumonia. This approach helps us to recognize not only the biological but also the various other factors that influence health.

Just as disease is caused by complex circumstances, so can a person's illness affect various other parts of his or her life. It is not hard

FIGURE 2-1.

A Hierarchy of Living Systems

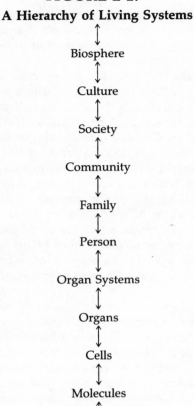

↑↓

Biosphere

↑↓

Culture

↑↓

Society

↑↓

Community

↑↓

Family

↑↓

Person

↑↓

Organ Systems

↑↓

Organs

↑↓

Cells

↑↓

Molecules

↑↓

to imagine how the respiratory therapist's pneumonia caused further disturbances at home and at the hospital, affecting not only his family but co-workers and patients and possibly their families.

Epidemiologist Leonard Sagan states:

> The unit of health must be broadened beyond the individual to include the entire social network on which the health of the individual depends; a healthy nation is more than a collection of healthy individuals. Just as no person is entirely self-contained ("no man is an island"), so too does the health of each of us depend upon those around us, upon the family, and also upon the larger network of a caring and nurturing community.[3]

Many chronic illnesses that are so prevalent today have far-reaching consequences. Arteriosclerosis, or hardening of the arteries, is a specific condition, but it can cause disease in a number of organs, such as the brain, kidneys, and heart. Illnesses that arise from this condition will affect an individual's functioning in the family and community.

As Howard Brody and David S. Sobel state in an article on "A Systems View of Health and Disease," in this model the effects of diseases are not revealed in a single organ or tissue but are seen as *"patterns of disruptions* manifested at various levels of the system at various times."[4] Even for individuals with the same diagnosis, this pattern will differ. Two people with coronary heart disease can have different risk factors for the disease. For instance, one may smoke and the other have high cholesterol, or one may be unable to cope with stress and the other get little exercise. Also, a person's illness will affect various levels of the hierarchy differently. One person's family may be very supportive and his social group may choose to deny his diagnosis, or he may be labeled by his culture as a "cardiac cripple." In other words, the pattern of cause and effect differs for each illness that an individual has and for each individual with that illness.

It is easy for a physician quickly to become overwhelmed by the implications of such a complex model of disease causation and treatment. Diagnosing complex interrelationships and causative factors is difficult. And besides, one cannot write a prescription for family harmony or financial security. But very often the physician is in a position to recognize the various potential causes and effects of an illness and can then either initiate intervention in those areas or suggest appropriate referrals.

This is a case in which an interdisciplinary health-care team, composed of medical, psychological, and spiritual practitioners, can address the concerns of the sick individual in an integrated manner. The members of the team are sensitive to the potential effects of the illness in the various areas of the person's life and they are able to help the person regain health or learn to cope with the disease in a manner that promotes wholeness.

For example, if our respiratory therapist had visited St. Luke Health Center when he had fallen ill, he would have seen the physician who would have diagnosed his illness and treated him appropriately. But the physician also would have asked him about his family, job, and other concerns in his life. In other words, the physician is interested in all significant levels of this person's hierarchy and wants to know: Why did you get sick now? The areas of distress in the therapist's life would become apparent after he answered the doctor's questions. Then the physician could offer some suggestions regarding the therapist's problems, or if the difficulties seemed more deep-seated, the physician might advise that the therapist seek counseling either alone or with his wife. The acute illness in this case, pneumonia, has brought attention to the fact that other disturbances exist in this person's life. By seeing a physician who is part of an interdisciplinary team, the respiratory therapist can be easily referred to a counselor who can address the therapist's areas of need beyond the purely physical. The physician and counselor work together closely and can exchange information about a person's difficulties and progress. A person treated by a team such as this receives integrated care and can become aware of the myriad of influences that contribute to health.

Illness involves every human dimension: physical, emotional, intellectual, social, and spiritual. Each individual person is also a system within himself or herself, with each dimension of the self interacting with every other dimension. And illness has implications for the individual in each of these human dimensions:

Physically, we need to look at the rate of wear and tear on the body (stress) and its internal and external sources, including health-risk factors, genetic predisposition, and infection.

Emotionally, we need to explore personal experience and feelings in order to make conscious our embodied beliefs.

Intellectually, we need to watch for symbolic meaning in the illness experience to shed light on other factors that may be present.

Socially, we need to pay close attention to changes in family and familylike social systems, and examine roles in these systems, including the impact of the illness on the family and the family's impact on the illness.

Spiritually, we need to examine our religious interpretation of the illness experience.

We resist the temptation to place these dimensions of human experience and illness experience in any sort of hierarchy. They are all very important in finding meaning in illness. Some, or all, of these elements may be involved in the onset of a particular illness; they are then all affected by the illness.

It is impossible to make generalizations about the meaning or experience of illness. Each person's experience of illness is unique. The health-care provider needs to be a reverent midwife to the process of allowing the meaning of an individual's illness to emerge.

As we proceed through the next section of this chapter, we pay particular attention to five major dimensions of the human person, each of which has an impact on the individual's illness experience.

Physical Dimension: Stress and Its Impact on Health

Stress may be described very simply as "the rate of wear and tear within the body," according to one definition by Hans Selye, a pioneer in psychosomatic medicine.[5] Wear and tear is increased dramatically with a physical reaction to an emergency, commonly called the "fight-or-flight" response. Nature intended the response to be temporary and life-protecting. However, many conditions in our society work together to make this response continuous and slowly, insidiously life-destroying.

Many experiences, both positive and negative, can be identified as stressors, or triggers of a physical reaction that increases wear and tear within the body. Marriage, job changes, vacation, a new home, a new baby, or retirement all present physical as well as emotional challenges. As long as one does not attempt to manage too many positive stressors at one time, an appropriate "gearing up" to meet a challenge is a harmless part of living a full life.

Environmental stressors, such as noise, air and water pollution, and general stressors, such as overcrowding in cities, deadline pressures, and competition, are the result of a complex social and economic structure that makes constant stress a way of life for most Americans. Certain beliefs, such as those behind workaholism, competition, materialism, or the need to earn love, drive a person from deep, unconscious layers of the psyche, and contribute to inordinate stress.

When the source of stress is clear, an individual may be better equipped to utilize a normal, adaptive stress reaction. However, when the source of stress is ambiguous or unconscious, or when there are too many sources of stress in a person's life at one time, the person is much more likely to exhibit a prolonged, potentially damaging stress reaction.

The fight-or-flight response may become habitual under prolonged, unabated stressful conditions. This response, which is appropriate in a crisis situation, can gradually become a way of life. This continuous reaction to stress can even become "normal" to the person who loses his or her sensitivity to changes in the body, who may even feel capable of adding *more* stress to his or her life. If this pattern persists, the sustained stress reaction begins to take a toll on the body, and often leads to one of the major stress-induced disorders: cardiovascular disease, arthritis, respiratory diseases, gastrointestinal problems, and allergies.

Case Study

Dorothy was a 53-year-old widow who had been employed as a secretary to a pastor for 12 years. The pastor had become ill during the previous year and was unable to fulfill his duties, so an assistant pastor was brought in temporarily. However, as the year progressed, the pastor's health deteriorated and it seemed very unlikely that he would ever return to his position. The assistant pastor took over more and more of the pastor's responsibilities and, three months prior to Dorothy's visit to St. Luke Health Center, he had hired his own administrative aide, a woman whom Dorothy described as very domineering.

During our visit with Dorothy, she expressed a fear of losing her job if the pastor retired and was replaced by the assistant. She also found it very difficult to work with the administrative aide who was usurping Dorothy's authority at every opportunity. Dorothy did not want to confront either the assistant pastor or his aide for fear that she would be fired on the spot. For the previous three weeks she had been experiencing morning headaches. She was concerned because she had high blood pressure, and although she was on medication, she worried that the blood pressure was not being controlled.

Dorothy appeared to be a very mild-mannered, soft-spoken woman. She told us that she rarely expressed anger and tried very hard to get along with people. She only wanted to do her job and feel that the church valued her service. When we took Dorothy's blood pressure, it was 196/114, alarmingly high. (Normal blood pressure is less than 140/90.) Two months before, Dorothy's blood pressure had been controlled with the medication she was taking.

During the visit, we asked Dorothy if she would try a relaxation exercise with us. She consented, and after 15 minutes of progressive muscle relaxation, we rechecked Dorothy's blood pressure. It had come down to 170/104—not normal, but certainly below what it had been. One month later, Dorothy returned to tell us that she had accepted a position in a neighboring city and would be moving soon. Her blood pressure had dropped to 150/80.

Dorothy's situation is not that unusual. We are all confronted daily with circumstances that cause us discomfort, both psychological and physical. We have come to call this discomfort "stress," and very often we accept it as a part of modern life. For some people, the discomfort progresses to actual disease or illness. But where does this stress reaction come from, and why do we react the way we do?

When we find ourselves in a dangerous or unpleasant situation, our bodies respond automatically so that we can better protect ourselves. Our adrenal glands, located on top of the kidneys, secrete hormones (adrenaline and noradrenaline) that circulate throughout the body and cause specific changes. Our heart rate speeds up, our blood pressure increases, pupils dilate, more blood goes to the muscles, and our breathing rate increases. These changes prepare our bodies either to fight the threat or to flee the situation, hence the term, fight-or-flight response. When the danger is gone, the body's functions return to the unalarmed state.

Perhaps you can recall a time when you or someone you love was involved in a dangerous situation, such as a fall, an encounter with a wild animal, or a car collision. Remember your heart pounding, the rapid breathing, the extraordinary speed, strength, and judgment that were available for the moment of crisis? Then, once the emergency situation was over, you probably experienced a feeling of tremendous relief.

This reaction is useful to us when we face an identifiable external threat to which we can respond rapidly. It turns out that we also react this way to a somewhat lesser degree when the unpleasant situation continues day after day, or when the threat is not external but is confined to our perceptions or beliefs. It is also influenced by whether or not we have a means of escape or the freedom to attack.

For example, Dorothy was confronted day after day with co-workers whom she did not trust and who devalued her work. She assumed, although she never confirmed it, that if she spoke up she would lose her job. For a long time, she felt that she needed to stay in her job out of loyalty to the pastor and out of fear of change.

In Dorothy's circumstances, as with many other people, this constant activation of the fight-or-flight response was translated into a chronic physical condition, high blood pressure. In addition to hypertension, chronic stress has also been associated with heart disease, headaches, peptic ulcers, asthma, arthritis, backaches, and rashes. Our bodies are not meant to be maintained in a perpetual state of alarm, but when this happens, various functions become altered and cause symptoms of disease. Unremitting stress also makes it difficult to maintain meaningful relationships, perform adequately at work, or just have fun. If we feel there are no ways to change a situation, we can become depressed. This emotional state can also lead to physical illness.

Continuous stress may sometimes cause a person to opt for illness as a way to be relieved temporarily of overwhelming responsibility. This is generally an unconscious decision, although occasionally people report making a conscious decision. If choosing illness seems to be the best option at a given moment, new strategies need to be learned as soon as possible.

Even physiological responses that were once thought to be beyond our control, such as breathing rate, temperature, heart rate, and blood pressure—all affected by the fight-or-flight response—have been convincingly demonstrated to be controllable in laboratory research. Biofeedback is helpful in detecting signs of chronic stress and teaching new patterns of response, particularly conscious relaxation.

Relaxation is not automatic, and certainly it is not as simple as taking a nap, watching television, or playing a game of tennis. Ironically, relaxation is something that most of us need to learn.

In chapter 6, we look at the different ways we can mitigate the effects of external threats (stressors) and how we can interrupt the fight-or-flight response when it is not needed. In chapters 3 and 4, we explore various spiritual disciplines that reduce many unnecessary internal stressors. Learning how to reduce stress, and how to react to stressful situations differently, can help prevent discomfort and disease.

Emotional Dimension: Emotions, Beliefs, and Health

Our bodies and our emotions are reliable communicators. They are able to "speak" truthfully to us about our situation, relationships, and events. The full range of emotions and physical responses make up a helpful language for our inner Selves to communicate with our conscious selves. Our bodies and emotions respond appropriately and automatically; we cannot stop this from occurring, but we are clearly conditioned to fight it.

"I shouldn't feel this way," we hear over and over again, as persons try to talk themselves out of their feelings, or to force themselves to forgive injuries without going through their anger and pain. Or, "I can understand why she acts that way," said by persons who take care of others' feelings while denying their own. Anger, aggression, the pain of loss, and sexual feelings are often unwelcome and vigorously denied. When we do not allow them, they do not go away:

they are stored in the body somewhere, to wait until we have grown into being able to face them (or until they lead to an illness, or possibly erupt unexpectedly in an act that seems "out of character").

A healthy body is resilient, according to philosopher Sam Keen. It surrenders to life and is flexible. A healthy body is able to respond, and has the ability to tense and to act forcefully when necessary, and the ability to relax completely. All of our emotions that were not allowed, all of our experiences that were too painful to deal with, all of the precious parts of our true Selves which felt unsafe are stored in the body, limiting its resilience and ability to respond, making it a little more vulnerable to injury or illness.[6] Another way of describing this phenomenon would be to say that patterns of physical response become habitual over time, such as muscular tension in the neck, and this limits the range of possible responses, such as relaxation, unless there is an actual emergency. The good news is that the limiting habits can be released and the range of possible responses can be increased through relearning relaxation and flexibility.

The use of biofeedback in our practice at St. Luke Health Center has revealed the sensitivity of the body to such subtle events as thoughts, words, images, emotions, or memories. Similarly, we have observed amazing physical responses to thoughts or words demonstrated through muscle testing: a positive thought, or a word such as "courage" actually strengthens a person, whereas a negative thought or word weakens the person significantly. Jeanne Achterberg states in her book, *Imagery in Healing*: "Every thought is accompanied by electrochemical change; that's what thinking is—electrochemical change."[7]

Similarly, bodywork such as Feldenkrais techniques or therapeutic massage has been regularly employed at St. Luke Health Center in conjunction with counseling because emotions and memories are frequently found to be released in the process of deep muscular relaxation or changes in body alignment.

Our entire personal histories and our beliefs are incarnate in our bodies. Sam Keen illustrates how every personal and corporate belief has an effect on our bodies. These may be religious beliefs, such as the notion that God is exclusively male, which can contribute to erect posture in proud men or sloping shoulders in defeated women, or the idea that body and spirit are separate, which can encourage a numbness and an alienation from devalued bodies. Corporate, political beliefs, such as the generally agreed-upon need for productivity, or the idea that time is money, often fuel an unhealthy drive to keep producing, no matter what the cost to other parts of one's life. Some beliefs become a part of us through advertising and mass media, such as the idea that we need more and more material possessions to be happy, to attain status, to be socially acceptable, or to find love. These beliefs can also drive persons with restless dissatisfaction. Medicine has affected our beliefs about, and experiences of, birth and death, making them something apart from life and nature and something to be feared, which causes us to resist them. Sometimes families share a worldview or form deeply held beliefs about individual family members that become self-fulfilling prophecies. Assigned gender roles affect posture and physical vulnerability: men in our culture are taught to hold back tears with rigidity in their chests; women often store tension in their shoulders to hold back their anger.[8]

At St. Luke Health Ministries, we would illustrate how our state of mental and physical health is determined by using an "iceberg model," based on the model by the same name offered in *Wellness Workbook*, by John W. Travis, MD, and Regina Sara Ryan.[9] An iceberg is an appropriate metaphor here because as impressive as these massive islands of ice are above the water, 90 percent of the mass is hidden below the water's surface. Similarly, a person's state of physical and mental health is like the portion of the iceberg that can be seen above the surface. Underneath that lie all the factors, experiences, and beliefs that influence our state of health: life-style and health habits, such as diet, exercise, use of seatbelts, and avoidance of alcohol and smoking; genetic makeup, personality, and attitudes; economics, culture, education, marital status, age, and gender; personal history; and worldview. Our worldview, or our beliefs about life, God, self, and others, is at the bottom of the iceberg, informing all of our other choices and experiences, and ultimately, our state of health.

Any disease—tension, workaholism, depression, sickness, or any form our illness may take—is a communication from one part of ourselves that attempts to tell us what we believe. We think we know what we believe, and these are our professed beliefs. However, there are always contradictions with our actual, *embodied* beliefs. I may profess to believe that rest is important and valuable while I live out a strongly held work ethic. If I contract a case of the flu and I feel relieved, that calls my attention to the discrepancy between my professed belief and my embodied belief. Do I need a medical excuse to allow myself to rest? Here is an opportunity to make a choice: will I make rest and recreation a priority in my life, or will I continue to become overworked and overtired, and get sick? If I want to enjoy my "down" time, it would be better for me to take a break when I'm feeling well.

Case Study

Mark came to St. Luke Health Center suffering from chronic, ulcerative colitis, with acute episodes when he was under stress. He was a gentle caregiver, a man who was always responsive to others' needs. He was a minister in an active church, a friend to many who depended on him, and also a graduate student. In addition, he held a part-time job to pay for graduate school, and was committed to his involvement in ACOA (Adult Children of Alcoholics). It was very clear to him and to us that his early experiences of neglect and deprivation as a child of abusive, alcoholic parents had formed a deep, core belief in him; "If I work real, real hard, maybe then I will be loved." His illness was so severe and had done so much damage that he had to have his colon surgically removed. The need to confront his belief behind his workaholism, to make significant changes in lifestyle, and to learn to take care of himself had reached the point where it was a matter of life and death. He chose life. There is no question that his decision requires extraordinary courage, as he struggles daily to learn to love and to take care of himself.

A life of self-sacrifice may require persons to look at their need to control their situation in order to protect themselves from vulnerability. Perfectionism may be a hard-driving attempt to earn love. Stress may be calling our attention to our slavery to time or to work.

Contradictions often exist between professed beliefs and embodied beliefs about God. For example, some people report that they believe that God is loving, while they are living out deep fear of God's judgment, or experiencing an inability to trust God and life, or feeling an urgent need to earn God's love.

Sam Keen teaches that the knots in our muscles cry out for us to look at what we are *not* allowing ourselves to feel, or to do, or to be. Knotted muscles are often a result of not allowing ourselves to feel or to express an emotion that we have judged to be unacceptable, such as anger, guilt, depression, or aggression. We can learn to allow ourselves to feel every emotion, trusting that our emotions are always reliable. Then we can simply observe what we feel, and choose an appropriate action or expression of that feeling. Denying our emotions is an attempt to avoid conflict. The problem is that it doesn't work:

our bodies and emotions take up the task of calling the conflict to our attention. People who swallow their anger, depression, guilt, and so on often get sick. No wonder some of "the nicest people" get sick.[10]

Another way that beliefs become embodied is through eidetic imagery, described by Akhter Ahsen as a powerful representation formed in a person's memory by significant events in his or her life. This image has three essential parts: a visual image, physical feelings, and a cognitive component.[11] These images are unearthed as health-care participants tell their personal experience of their illness. These may be graphic images of the experience of illness, such as falling apart, being crushed, feeling torn, or having deep feelings of abandonment, fear, betrayal, helplessness, and so on. Typically the bottom line in most of our illness is a preverbal sense of being unlovable, unworthy, or unable to trust. The eidetic images that promote illness become available for transformation into health-promoting images through counseling and prayer. For example, a Christian who discovers the image of a beaten, abandoned part of himself or herself, may find healing in praying with Jesus' parable of the Good Samaritan.[12] The wounded part of one's self can be cared for by one's inner Good Samaritan, the true Self, or Christ within.

Unconscious beliefs are particularly potent in our lives. Staying stuck in our illness can be an unconscious attempt to avoid our deeper conflicts, or a fear of facing our true Selves. If that is the case, then the suffering of our illness will become greater than the legitimate suffering it attempts to avoid. On the other hand, illness can be a way to identify our deeper conflicts and resolve them, to face ourselves and become whole. The choice is ours.

Social Dimension: Illness within the Family System

Rabbi and family therapist, Dr. Edwin H. Friedman, describes emotional processes at work within the family and familylike systems in his book, *Generation to Generation*. These emotional processes, including interdependence, the need for equilibrium, and the roles individuals play within the family network, all have an impact on the physical, emotional, and spiritual well-being of family members.[13]

Just as the human body is made up of distinct organs and organ systems, the human family is made up of individuals and emotional networks. Just as organs within the human body are adversely affected by the overfunctioning, underfunctioning, or dysfunctioning of other organs—for example, underfunctioning kidneys can leave salts circulating in the body that contribute to heart disease—so also, illness may be a signal of a problem within a family system. The problem may well be in the system, rather than simply in one of its parts.

Every person is born into a family of origin; many adults marry and create new families. We have extended families, and familylike emotional networks in the workplace, school, church, and community. When we speak of family in the context of health care, we mean any system of human relationships that functions as a unit, whether it is a biological family, or any other emotional network made up of persons who are not biologically related.

The experience of family is a powerful determining factor in sickness and health. For our understanding of some of the dynamics of illness and health, it is important to include a brief overview of the family system and its impact on health at this point in our discussion. We discuss healthy families and the healing potential of relationships further in chapter 8.

One of the fundamental principles of family, according to Friedman, is that any relational network seeks equilibrium. It can do this in ways that are healthy or unhealthy; stability is more important to family than how that stability is to be achieved. One can imagine a family system as being much like a hanging mobile: when one part is rocked, the whole mobile is set in motion; the movement decreases until balance is restored. Similarly, when one person changes in a family, this change affects everyone else; equilibrium is thrown off, and every effort is made to return to smooth functioning. The family system generally does not like to be unstable, so it tends to resist change.

The individual who seeks medical attention for a physical or emotional health problem may be identified within his or her family as "the sick one." Very often, this person is not "the sick one" at all, but rather, this is the one in whom a family problem surfaces.

Illness in one family member can stabilize a family, taking the focus of attention away from an unresolved issue within the family. This is an effective, unconscious technique of maintaining balance within the family. If true healing is to take place, the family issue needs to be dealt with; otherwise the symptoms recycle to another family member or recur within the same person.

The physician or counselor at St. Luke Health Center who was the first contact for a health-care participant would ask questions to find out what was happening in one's family system(s) that disrupted the balance to produce discomfort at that time. Three common situations are often factors in the onset of illness (Edwin Friedman calls them "malignant family positions"): an intense emotional triangle between family members, a disturbance in a deeply dependent relationship, and self-sabotage.

The first situation, that of an emotional triangle, occurs when two persons have an uncomfortable relationship, or an unresolved issue between them. This issue or discomfort is avoided by focusing attention on a third person or issue; for example, a couple focuses on a son's alcoholism to avoid issues within their marital relationship. Another common type of triangle occurs when one person tries to change the relationship between two others, such as a woman who involves herself in the relationship between a co-worker and their boss. Triangles can occur within a nuclear family, or within multigenerational extended families, and with persons who are living or dead.

In the second situation, when two or more persons are intertwined in a deeply dependent relationship, any change in any person becomes a crisis of sorts. The others in this type of family system automatically react: they may feel the same way as the person who changes (if you're down, I'm down; if you're up, I'm up), or they may compensate (if you're down, I'll take over for you; if you're up, I'm down). Each person's actions and feelings are determined by the actions and feelings of others, rather than by their own unique experience and needs.

One of the most frightening disturbances in overly dependent relationships happens when one person in the relationship begins to become more authentically himself or herself. The more dependent the relationship, the more panic and resistance results in the person who is not ready to change. The issue may surface in the form of a physical problem, an emotional problem, or a social problem *in any family member*.

To use an example common to the 1980s—if a woman who has submerged her needs and her identity in taking care of her family begins to identify her own needs and act on them, creating a separate life for herself while remaining firmly connected with the family, the rest of her family will be challenged to adapt. A deeply dependent family has difficulty handling change and stress, so a symptom, any symptom, may appear in her husband, any one of her children, or even the woman herself.

As health-care practitioners, we cannot make any assumptions about the person who presents himself or herself with an illness of

some sort. We may be working with the family member most motivated to change, and who needs our support to face ongoing resistance from the family system. Or we may be working with a very
resistant family member who is invested in remaining ill, or at least
in maintaining the status quo within the family.

The third family dynamic situation that can be a factor in disease
causation is that of self-sabotage. This sometimes occurs when a person who has been enmeshed in a deeply dependent system has made
some significant strides in taking responsibility for her or his own
actions and feelings. The person then does something self-defeating,
or becomes ill, rather than risk success, which would require dying
to an old self-image and allowing a new one to be born.

The illness experience takes place in a web of relationships that not
only affects the onset and the course of illness, but is profoundly
affected by the illness as well. An illness may bring a family or other
social network together into deeper relationship, more support, and
better communication than ever before, or an illness can be a source
of overwhelming suffering, grief, burden, or frustration to a family.
Each practitioner must listen carefully to the participant's interpretation of his or her illness experience, especially regarding its place
in relationships. The message of Dr. Kleinman in *The Illness Narratives*
speaks directly to those who seek to address the illness as well as the
disease:

> Illness is not simply a personal experience; it is transactional, com-
> municative, profoundly social. The study of illness meanings is not
> only about one particular individual's experience; it is also very much
> about social networks, social situations, and different forms of social
> reality. Illness meanings are shared and negotiated. They are an integral
> dimension of lives lived together. . . an inquiry into the meanings of
> illness is a journey into relationships.[14]

What we have said about illness and the family applies to other
social groups that function as a unit as well. It is clear that the cultural
family, the church family, the work family, the human family, and
the global family all have an impact on the physical, emotional, and
spiritual well-being of individuals, and vice versa. For example, we
cannot overlook the irresponsibility in work settings where people
are exposed to occupational hazards, or the serious dysfunction in
church families where persons are socialized to accept limitations on
their wholeness. Relationships that hurt and relationships that heal
are studied further in chapter 8.

Intellectual Dimension: Symbolic Meaning of Illness

As the layers of experience in an individual's illness are discovered one by one, much like peeling away layers of an onion, a theme will often emerge. Patterns repeat themselves. Some say these are the lessons we need to learn in our lifetime, and the lesson is patiently repeated as often as we need it until we grow into the ability to resolve the situation in a creative, life-giving way.

At St. Luke Health Center, we have frequently observed that the themes that surface in persons who are courageous far travelers on the spiritual journey are typically present in some aspect of their illness experience. A person who experiences the emptiness of present-day loss combined with early childhood experiences of being unloved or unwanted may find the void being filled with cancer. The early experience of extreme childhood restrictions may be repeated in adulthood as environmental illness, an allergy to almost everything. A person who chronically feels unsupported may also suffer chronic back pain. Overweight persons very often feel unsafe at a core level. Rigidity, control, or stubbornness are frequently embodied in a stiff neck; anger often lurks in aching shoulders. The correspondences we have observed between symptoms and deeper meanings are not absolute truths, but they do suggest clues about an individual's core issues.

The symptom may be a symbol, that is, a representation of an abstract concept. Conversely, the abstract idea becomes a physical reality when the symbol becomes incarnate as a symptom. The question of whether certain personality traits, core beliefs, or life issues correspond with particular diseases and target organs is a lively issue. Controlled research has yielded conflicting results.

Bernie Siegel articulates the insight of many competent, scientific clinicians when he states:

> Target organs—parts of the body with special significance to the conflicts or losses in a person's life—are the most likely areas for the disease to take root. Franz Alexander, the father of psychosomatic medicine, recognized this over 40 years ago when he wrote: "There is much evidence that, just as certain pathological organisms have a specific affinity for certain organs, so also certain emotional conflicts possess specificities and accordingly tend to afflict certain internal organs."[15]

Siegel also reports on the extensive longitudinal study by Dr. Caroline Bedell Thomas, begun in 1946, which followed over 1300 medical students yearly for decades after their graduation. One totally un-expected finding was that persons who were restricted in expressing emotion had a very high incidence of cancer, and that Thomas could predict the target organ based on the drawings they had done as medical students as a minor part of the battery of tests.[16] Similarly, research being done on the neurological link between mind and body is producing a growing body of evidence that the limbic system of the brain, which is also the processing center of emotions, the hy-pothalamus, which is linked with the immune system, and the pi-tuitary, do in fact target certain organs in response to feeling states. Jeanne Achterberg gives a highly readable account of current research in her book, *Imagery in Healing*.[17]

On the other hand, recent meta-analysis by Drs. H. Friedman and S. Booth-Kewley of over 100 smaller studies demonstrated a link be-tween the neurotic personality and disease in general, rather than linking specific traits with specific target organs or specific illnesses. The neurotic personality is characterized by chronic anxiety, sadness, tension, hostility, and/or depression. Friedman and Booth-Kewley believe other studies may have failed because they tended to be too specific in studying a particular isolated personality trait, but the combined pool of thousands of subjects showed a clear pattern: neu-rotic persons become sick more often with a variety of illnesses.[18]

The validity of lists linking traits and issues with target organs and diseases is arguably questionable from a scientific point of view. How-ever, we do not want to throw out the baby with the bathwater: the lists can be extremely helpful even if they are not absolute. For ex-ample, Louise Hay's list in her book, *You Can Heal Your Life*,[19] may seem too pat to be taken seriously, but there can be no real harm in asking one's self if the issues named there could possibly be relevant. At the very least, these lists may be used as a reference point, to which one might respond "that's not exactly it for me, it's more like. . . . "

Case Study

Carolyn was going through a period of transition in her life, from talking about writing to actually doing it, from demanding equality to becoming equal, from stuffing negative feelings to owning them and expressing them. Overwhelmed with change, and bogged down in a major writing project with a deadline rapidly approaching, she noticed herself clearing her throat all the time, and sometimes when she opened her mouth to speak, her voice was not there. The croaking, clearing, and coughing persisted for weeks, at a minor irritation level. Her physician diagnosed it as a lingering aftereffect of the flu she had contracted some months earlier, and expressed confidence that it would clear up by itself. When she looked her symptom up on Hay's list, just to prove that such generalizations are oversimplified, she read:

> The throat represents our ability to "speak up" for ourselves, to "ask for what we want," to say "I am," etc. . . . The throat also represents the creative flow in the body. This is where we express our creativity; and when our creativity is stifled and frustrated, we often have throat problems. . . . The energy center in the throat, the fifth chakra, is the place in the body where change takes place. When we are resisting change or are in the middle of change or are trying to change, we often have a lot of activity in our throats.[20]

Caroline concluded that Louise Hay must have been reading her journal.

It is important to remember that working with an illness on a symbolic level is in no way a substitute for medical attention to the physical problem. Medical care is appropriate and necessary; identifying and resolving the issues revealed at the symbolic level is complementary. The two approaches together can bring about healing that lasts; either one alone is generally inadequate, and omitting medical care can be downright dangerous.

Spiritual Dimension: Religious Interpretations of Suffering

In our human need for meaning, especially in times of illness or loss, people often grab onto handy religious interpretations of their experience of suffering. The most common religious interpretations we heard at St. Luke Health Center include:

"Why did God send this misfortune?" (i.e., God is responsible.)

"Sickness is a form of correction by our loving God." (i.e., I am being punished for sin, or if I had lived correctly, I would not be in this predicament.)

"God gives suffering to favored children to draw them into a deeper faith relationship." (Thanks, but no thanks.)

Illness and loss are difficult enough to bear, but each of these commonly held ideas contributes to a great deal of unnecessary additional suffering. As an identified Christian healing ministry, we at St. Luke Health Center believed that we were in a unique position to respond to human suffering in a way that was compassionate, liberating, and nonjudgmental. Our Christianity gave us and those who came to us a point of reference. We did not attempt to make converts; we wanted to set people free.

To those who felt that God is somehow responsible for human suffering, we would call to mind the example of Jesus, whose ministry is characterized by a commitment to healing. Everywhere Jesus went, he touched, healed, forgave, set free, exorcised demons, and restored sight, hearing, mobility, even life itself. He was clearly opposed to anything that limited people's experience of fullness of life and personal relationship with God. God's will for us is revealed in Jesus' ministry: healing and abundant life. If we are to follow his example, we are not to settle for less for ourselves or for those who seek our help.

The question of the relationship between sickness and sin has been around for aeons. In contemporary secular language, it may be framed as illness as a consequence of straying from the path of wholeness. Jesus addressed this issue when his disciples asked him about why a particular man was born blind, "Rabbi, who sinned, this man or his parents, for him to have been born blind?" Jesus responded, "Neither he nor his parents sinned; he was born blind so that the works of God might be displayed in him."[21] Again, Jesus spoke very directly about suffering as punishment:

> Do you suppose that the Galileans who suffered like that were greater sinners than any other Galileans? They were not, I tell you. . . . Or those eighteen on whom the tower at Siloam fell and killed them: Do you suppose that they were more guilty than all the other people living in Jerusalem? They were not, I tell you.[22]

Clearly, those who are sick or injured are no better or worse than those who are well. In a like manner, we are all called to respond to illness with skill and compassion and *without judgment*.

The notion of illness leading people into a deeper relationship with God, or how good things often come out of an illness, as supporting the idea that sickness is a gift from a loving God is ludicrous. Yes, sometimes good things do come out of an illness, but that is a retrospective insight and a sign of God's goodness that everything is redeemable: it does not mean that illness is inherently good. Are we to allow people to continue to suffer because it is God's gift to them? Can you picture a loving parent giving a beloved child the gift of a little cancer or depression so the parent and child can have quality time together in the course of illness? Can you imagine Jesus telling the sick and crippled people who came to him in throngs, "Stay sick, and thank God for this special blessing?" He did not do that, and neither should we.

We cannot answer the question, "Where is God in this experience?" *for* anyone else; rather, we must be willing to *be with* others in their experience as they live with the questions and wait for their personal answers to emerge. This "being with" is at the heart of health care. As Arthur Kleinman writes in *The Illness Narratives*: "Legitimating the patient's illness experience—authorizing that experience, auditing it empathetically—is a key task in the care of the chronically ill. . . . "[23] Being with a sick person, without judgment, creates space for meaning to emerge and for the holy to be revealed.

As we travel through layers of meaning on the inward journey, whether on our own journeys or as privileged listeners to others, we often arrive at a deep level of core belief, or core feeling, or core image that needs to be healed. This deep experience might sometimes be described in spiritual terms as an experience of evil, a consequence of another's destructiveness, or a need for deliverance from a demonic, or destructive spirit; or it may be described in psychological terms as possession by an archetype or a complex, or an internalized oppressor. Either way, persons attempt to describe an experience of a powerful alien movement within themselves that seems to have a life and a personality of its own, which is not in keeping with a sense of "true Self," or the person we have been created to be. Arriving at a place of knowing and naming this destructive "other" within one's self is a remarkable achievement, but insight and willpower alone do not bring freedom. At this point, we must acknowledge our dependence on God. Articulating our specific need in prayer reflects our readiness for healing, and opens the way to receive the healing we seek.

God is present in the healing process in many ways: suffering with us in our brokenness, calling us to wholeness, waiting for us to seek healing, empowering us for the journey toward wholeness, and healing us when we are open to receive new life. (Please remember that we are talking about healing at this point, regardless of whether or not curing the disease takes place.)

Each person who served as a staff member at St. Luke Health Center shares a belief in Something, Someone beyond ourselves, whom we name God, which is actively involved in every aspect of the healing journey. We believe because each of us has experienced the Holy ourselves, touching our own lives at deep, broken, growing edges. We believe because we have been privileged witnesses to grace at work in the lives of persons who came to us for help. We believe because we each offer ourselves as willing channels of God's healing energy for others, and both we and those for whom we pray experience healing as a result. We know ourselves well enough to know that we are truly "earthen vessels"—cracked and chipped, but usable—as Paul wrote in his second letter to the Corinthians: "We are only the earthenware jars that hold this treasure, to make it clear that such an overwhelming power comes from God and not from us" (2 Cor. 4:7).

IMPLICATIONS FOR HEALTH CARE PROVISION

Our experience at St. Luke Health Center completely confirms Arthur Kleinman's assertion that healing requires attention to the illness experience as well as control of the disease. Illness has many meanings: it means something different to the suffering individual, to that person's family, to the health-care providers, and to the larger community. Attending the illness experience, watching for its meanings in a particular situation, requires valuing the person's report of their illness experience, as well as test results, physical examination, X rays, and so on.

Finding meaning in each unique case requires reverent attention, patient waiting; meaning cannot be rushed or imposed prematurely. Any preconceived notions about the meaning of illness does psychological and spiritual violence to the suffering individual. Meaning comes through the experience and reflection of the person who is ill, not necessarily from the knowledge of the health-care provider. The health-care provider serves by creating space for reflection and facilitating the process.

In order to provide health care that enhances finding meaning, the physician must be priest/shaman as well as doctor, or else he or she must be assisted by an interdisciplinary team. Since unconscious concepts are powerful in influencing our sickness and health, the team should include persons who are gifted at facilitating bringing the unconscious to the light of conscious awareness. There are many valuable techniques for accessing this information, for example, bodywork, or working with dreams or drawings. The images can then be brought to counseling and prayer.

Health care is always rooted in a belief system. Health-care providers need to be aware of the belief system that underlies their approach. Conventional health care services often flow from an unarticulated faith in technology, medical science alone, and bodies as mechanical wonders separate from mind and spirit. This model does an excellent job of treating disease, but it is severely limited in addressing the human need to find meaning in the experience of illness, or even providing lasting cures. Being clear about what is offered allows the highly motivated patient to seek out supplementary services to address other contributing factors.

Alternatively, offering health care as ministry rooted in a traditional faith has numerous advantages: when the faith tradition is shared by providers and participants, we meet on common ground; when it is not shared, it still offers meaning to the provider and a reference point for the participant. Our participants at St. Luke Health Center did not need to share our beliefs in order to benefit from our belief. The mere fact that we were rooted in a solid tradition could be a stabilizing, anchoring experience for persons whose lives were affected by illness. As an identified Christian healing ministry, the staff of St. Luke Health Center was able to offer a lifeline of hope to persons who might otherwise suffer needlessly from the additional difficulty of being lost and rudderless in a meaningless sea of overwhelming experiences.

IMPLICATIONS FOR PREVENTIVE HEALTH CARE

Life includes the possibility of disease, even if a person does all the "right" things. Within the order of the cosmos, there seems to be an element of randomness. Within the wonder and complexity of our bodies and minds, there is the possibility of natural disasters in the form of disease. Within the interconnectedness of all of creation, there is room for collective responsibility for one another's disease. We do not hold individuals responsible for causing their own disease or for curing themselves; however, paradoxical as it may seem, we do believe that much disease is preventable, and that individuals can actively minimize their chances of becoming sick.

A personal program of disease prevention should include attention to one's inner, spiritual life; healthy life-style, including good nutrition, exercise, moderation, and safety practices; stress management; integrity in family and other personal relationships; creativity, and service to others. Spiritual disciplines create space in our lives to contemplate, to find meaning, to become aware of embodied beliefs, to listen to the Holy within us and around us. Good health habits enhance immunity and safety; stress management reduces unnecessary wear and tear. Good communication and care of relationships provide mutual support, opportunity for growth and transformation, and the social environment needed for good health. Creative work, service to others, caring for the environment, raising families, and similar endeavors allow us to express the gift we have been created to be. Each of these elements of a personal preventive health-care program is discussed in more detail in later chapters of this book.

Staying well, like getting well, requires learning to honor one's own inner wisdom, to trust one's Self. No one can define healing, transformation, conversion, vocation, or meaning for someone else. The answers for *you* are within *you*, as guided by God's own Spirit. What do you feel? What do you need? What do you value? What motivates you? What is your experience? What is your prayer for yourself?

As you read these questions, you may feel them to be uncomfortably self-centered. By far the vast majority of people have been taught, directly or indirectly, that if they are themselves no one will love them, or that human beings are naturally sinful and selfish. It is often a difficult and frightening path to learn to trust one's Self and to trust the gracefulness of life, but trust can be learned, one day at a time, one step at a time.

Any person, any experience that told you that you are not lovable, or that you are not good enough, lied to you. The Book of Consolation (Isa. 40–55) is overflowing with assurances of God's infinite goodness and love. Spending time with its words and images can transform your sense of self, enabling you to re-member, to reconnect with the originally blessed creature you are. We have been told:

> for the mountains may depart,
> the hills be shaken,
> but my love for you will never leave you
> and my covenant of peace with you will never be shaken,
> says YHVH who takes pity on you. (Isa. 54:10)

> Do not be afraid, for I have redeemed you;
> I have called you by your name, you are mine.
> Should you pass through the sea, I will be with you;
> or through rivers, they will not swallow you up.
> Should you walk through fire, you will not be scorched
> and the flames will not burn you.
> For I am YHVH, your God,
> the Holy One of Israel, your savior. . . .

Because you are precious in my eyes,
because you are honored and I love you, . . .
Do not be afraid, for I am with you. (Isa. 43:1–5)

Scripture assures us that each person is personally known and loved by our Creator, that we share in God's own nature, and that the truth of who we are is love. People who learn to let in God's love are able to put down their defenses and to trust. Undefended, unconflicted persons are actually very generous as goodness flows freely from the center of their being. Our true Selves are trustworthy.

In order to get in touch with the true Self, we have to create space in our busy, noisy lives to listen to the still, small voice of God within. The next chapter, on spiritual disciplines, gives suggestions on how we might do this.

3

Creating Space for the Holy

"Spiritual life" affects every part of our lives and health—work, relationships, hobbies, politics, priorities. Spirit is embodied in flesh—our flesh. Spirituality is made up of everyday occurrences, the joys and irritations of daily living: sharing the bathroom, listening to children, dealing with the boss, driving in traffic, spending money.

Too often we think of "spiritual life" as set apart—an hour or two in church on Sunday, time set aside for prayer and Scripture study, lives set apart in monasteries. This overlooks the spiritual dimension of everyday life: where is God in the moment-to-moment interactions of parenting, marriage, workplace, traffic, school?

SPIRIT AND DISCIPLINE

God is in all of creation, and all of creation is in God. The idea of God and spirit as "other" or "out there" apart from the natural, physical world is a dangerous, potent form of dualism. Matter and spirit, time and eternity, coexist as dimensions of reality, here and now.

The great scholar and expert on mythology, Joseph Campbell, describes spirit as the "bouquet of life," a fragrance emanating out of life.[1] Spirit is the life principle that we share with all other persons, with God and with all of creation. The spiritual journey is a process of liberation, an unfolding, much like the petals of a flower gracefully and naturally unfold, as the human spirit is set free to discover union with the universal Spirit, which we call God.

"Spiritual life" is not a separate little compartment in one's life or psyche or schedule; it is *how we live* our lives. The conscious life of the spirit leads to unity; denying or restricting conscious spiritual life leads to alienation. Through openly facing life's challenges, and facing ourselves honestly, we gradually discover the truth of at-one-ment with God, with our true Selves, with others, with nature, and with the work of human hands. To live and grow in this truth *is* spiritual growth.[2]

The path of spiritual growth is indeed "the road less traveled," according to author and psychiatrist M. Scott Peck. This business of living the truth requires discipline, hard work, and pain; it requires giving up precious illusions, security, judgments, and false pride. The rewards are great, however, and the freedom, empowerment, and union that result from living the truth make it worth the effort.[3]

Discipline involves facing what is, confronting legitimate pain, staying at the task, taking responsibility, and delaying gratification. All of this requires flexibility, judgment, and effort. Self-discipline demands much, and the willingness to expend the effort is truly a manifestation of love.[4]

Spiritual growth does not come naturally. It takes training and vigilance to face into the challenge of living truthfully, because facing reality often requires the pain of loss. Our instincts are to flee or to resist pain. These losses involve letting go of control; giving up precious, but inaccurate, images of ourselves; facing the reality of our relationships with parents, spouse, children, or God; giving up unrealistic expections; accepting our mortality and other hard realities of existence.[5]

Spiritual disciplines are those practices that help us to overcome our fight-or-flight instincts when confronted with possible pain. It requires a mature, conscious decision to face the pain of spiritual growth, a decision based on the inner knowledge that the pain of growth is less than the pain of resistance and its resulting diminishment of life. In order to enjoy abundant life, we freely choose the path of discipline, which is also the path of love.

Conscious spiritual life is disciplined life, which empowers those who practice it, and deepens their commitment to love the people and the world around them. As Evelyn Underhill wrote in *Practical Mysticism*, spiritual life is not a special career, apart from the physical world, but is an essential part of becoming a complete human being. Its function, and its practicality, lies in that it will

increase, not diminish, the total efficiency, the wisdom and steadfast-
ness, of those who try to practise it. It will help them to enter, more
completely than ever before, into the life of the group to which they
belong.[6]

Spiritual life is clearly practical when we consider our use of time.
Time is the medium in which we live our lives, make our decisions,
forge our relationships. How might we experience the holy in everyday life?

TIME MANAGEMENT AS SPIRITUAL DISCIPLINE[7]

"I have to run."
"Where has the time gone?"
"I don't have time to waste."
"I have too much time on my hands."

Such statements reveal our attitude toward time and our sense of
personal power: Do I see time as enemy or friend? Does time have
control over my life or am I in control of my use of time? Is my time
obsessively focused on tasks, or uselessly frittered away, or flexible?
    Classical Greek thinking identified two kinds of time: *chronos*, which
refers to measurable duration of time; and *kairos*, which refers to a
special moment, a "right" time of unusual religious significance.
These notions of time reveal two very different ways of experiencing
the *same* time.
    We may simply experience time as *chronos*—minutes, hours, days,
weeks, months, years in history. In Jewish and Christian traditions,
God enters human history and human relationships. The historical
events of the Jewish people shape their religious tradition: their experiences of bondage in Egypt, the Exodus, the rule of David, the
destruction of the Temple and other historical events are powerful,
universal metaphors of personal and collective spiritual journey. In
the Christian tradition, God enters history in the person of Jesus. The
events of his life describe the universal call to triumph over darkness
and destruction through faithful living, dying to self, redemption,
and Resurrection. The events of our lives connect with these universal
images. The images, in turn, enable us to interpret our experiences
in light of a larger religious story, which results in meaning. In the
history of humanity, and in our individual, personal histories, God
meets us in chronological time.

Paradoxically, God is experienced by many as *beyond* history. The mystical traditions in every major faith seek direct encounter with God, who is outside of time, existing before and after creation. Therefore, we may also experience time as *kairos*, as well as chronological. This is not an either/or proposition, but a realization of the potential in time to meet God-who-is-beyond-time. A *kairos* moment is an opening into the sacred, the timeless, the infinite, and has been described as a peak experience, as mystical or unitive experience, as breakthrough, or as a moment when time seemed suspended. It is a moment of truth, in which we experience the Infinite, *which was there all along*.[8]

Any experience can be a *kairos* moment, even illness. Just as Jacob wrestled with God until daybreak, and then would not let him go until he received a blessing,[9] illness can be a time of encounter with God, struggle, and blessing. Jungian analyst Roger Woolger describes this paradoxical experience as a "dark night, full of the light of God and dark struggle, forged into union in the fire of suffering."[10] Whatever our experience, the invitation is to enter it fully, expecting to meet God there.

To see how our time can be experienced as kairotic as well as chronological, let us examine some of the attitudes and behaviors that make time *un*holy. What cuts us off from experiencing the sacred in our lives?

Excessive Busy-ness. The frantic pace of modern life subjects us to its innate violence and gradually destroys communication with our true Selves and God within. It is quite possible to enjoy the misery of being far too busy and hardly notice that God has been crowded out of the picture.

Our busy-ness may simply be an attempt to prove to ourselves and to others that we really are important. Work can be an addiction that helps us avoid troubling feelings, or coming to terms with ourselves. The best way to find out what our busy-ness does for us is to stop being so busy and to observe carefully what feelings surface in us.[11]

Developing Exits. Exits are the ways we avoid painful situations, particularly in relationships. Activities, such as working, engaging in hobbies, fantasizing, watching TV, entertaining, cleaning, sleeping, reading, engaging in sex, or eating, are exits only if we use them to avoid someone or something.[12] The best way to uncover our hidden motivations is to ask ourselves what would happen if we gave up a certain activity.

Responding to Every Need That Presents Itself. We cannot be all things to all persons, but some of us sure try. This apparent generosity is actually a lack of trust. When we feel we must respond to every need, we are not trusting God to provide for human needs, and we are not trusting others to pick up their share of responsibility. Actions motivated by a compulsive sense of responsibility ("I have to do this"), if frequent, are likely to result in fatigue, anger, frustration, and burnout. Saying "no" to some requests allows us to say "yes" to our own vocation and unburdens us of the weight of overresponsibility.[13]

Allowing One's Life to Get Out of Balance. A well-balanced life includes work, recreation, prayer, family time, solitude, time with friends, exercise, service, time spent outdoors, and so on. A life of frantic activity cuts us off from the wisdom of God within us; a life of prayer without service is stillborn; a too-active social life may keep us from facing ourselves in solitude; the work ethic may prevent us from experiencing the renewal of play. An unbalanced life is unwhole and unholy.

Seeing Time as an Enemy. This may reflect an unconscious view that time leads one closer and closer to death, which results in compulsive combat against the natural process of aging. One might instead appreciate the maturity and seasoning that is possible only with the passage of time.

Also, time may seem to be an enemy if one sees spiritual life as exclusively outside of time and as separate from the material world. If we are open to experiencing the Holy in time, then time becomes an opportunity and a friend.[14]

Feeling My Time Is Not My Own. Seeing one's self as a victim of endless demands, expectations, and responsibilities that come from outside of one's self denies our ability to make choices about our use of time. It calls for serious, prayerful reflection on what one is truly called to do and to be. This can be done most honestly with the help of a trusted friend, a spiritual director, or a therapist.

Most people engage in some of these behaviors at least some of the time. Rather than becoming discouraged, we can look at ourselves compassionately and forgive ourselves for not knowing the best way to care for ourselves. We will experience less pain and greater reward in the long run if we are willing to embrace the path of discipline and love.

People who pay attention to the single activity before them at any given moment frequently find that their energy and attention are not fragmented. They are able to do one thing at a time, and let go of whatever is undone. They are able to accomplish more than they expect because no energy has been wasted on worrying about "too much to do, too little time."

Time is not our master, but our servant—a gift from God for us to use. Those with an attitude of abundance will find that time multiplies like the Gospel story of the loaves and fishes: the time will be there for everything that we truly need to do and that we are called to do. Time pressure is usually a symptom that we are trying to do too much, or are taking on too much responsibility.

How can we take responsibility for our use of time and structure it in a way that creates space for the holy, in order to make life-giving choices about life-style, health habits, and relationships?

ENCOUNTERING THE SPIRITUAL REALM

Experiences of the Infinite result in the conviction that there is "more to life than meets the eye." We might experience the Holy unexpectedly and spontaneously in *kairos* moments such as:

Connecting deeply with another person

Being profoundly moved by a work of art or musical performance

Beholding the vastness and wonder of nature

Facing awesome power, such as the ocean or a rocket launch.

In such moments, it seems as if the veil that conceals the infinite has quietly slipped away, and the truth and unity are revealed. The vision or presence in that unitive moment shatters our conceptions of life with its comfortable limits, illusions, and separation. These moments of truth change us— temporarily, or permanently. We are unprepared for the bliss of life without limits, so the veil that separates us from paradise returns. But we remember our "unitive glimpses," and know that Jesus' teaching is true: the reign of God is *now*.

Spiritual disciplines allow us to encounter the Holy, beyond intellectualization, religious doctrines, or preconceived images. Opening ourselves to the Divine Mystery requires that we increase our attentiveness to the Holy, and relinquish control to allow ourselves to be changed.

We make contact with the Infinite Source of all power and illumination through:

Our own unconscious

Revelation of the Holy through other persons or through human expression, such as the humanities, the spoken word, law, and so on

The ongoing revelation of the Creator through all of creation, from atomic particles to the cosmos.

We live in the physical world and the spiritual world simultaneously: our senses are windows to the physical world around us; our minds open to the spiritual world that permeates and encompasses the physical world.

To those who question the existence of the nonphysical, spiritual realm, we cannot offer scientific "proof." We can point to dreams, visions, revelation, healing, wisdom, inspiration, prophecy, and experiences of angels, demons, deceased persons, and spirit guides, as direct experiences of powerful nonphysical realities that occur in the lives of many persons, and are described in religious literature of every major faith tradition. In his book, *Companions on the Inner Way*, Morton Kelsey describes 36 varieties of distinguishable spiritual experience, and goes on to say that spiritual experience is so prevalent that one would have to make a deliberate effort in order to avoid this dimension of reality.[15]

In chapter 2, we presented a systems approach to understanding illness, which showed the individual in the middle of a hierarchy of interactive levels. Similarly, we can think of the individual as part of another highly interactive system that includes the spiritual dimension of life, both in the physical world and the nonphysical realm.

Figure 3-1 illustrates the relationship of the individual to the infinite in the physical and nonphysical worlds. This representation is nonhierarchical, but circular: the Alpha and Omega is God. Figure 3-2 explains the terms used in Figure 3-1. Divine life—truth and energy—flows freely and inexhaustibly through every available channel, to every level of consciousness. We can encounter the Holy within ourselves and outside of ourselves, and be changed, enlightened, and empowered.

Spiritual life and energy flow in a circle from God within us to God around us and in other persons and back again, depending on our openness. We can erect barricades to spiritual life flowing through us through busy-ness, unfinished emotional work, resistance, or any number of ways. God is available through countless sources. For those interested in deepening their understanding of the relationship be-

FIGURE 3-1.

A Systems Approach to Spiritual Realities

Outer World

Inner World

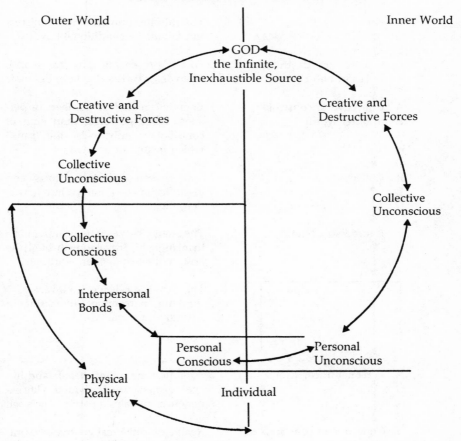

Note: Each level of energy and consciousness is able to interact with every other level of energy and consciousness, without having to flow through all the other levels along the way.

FIGURE 3-2.

Terms Used in "A Systems Approach to Spiritual Realities"

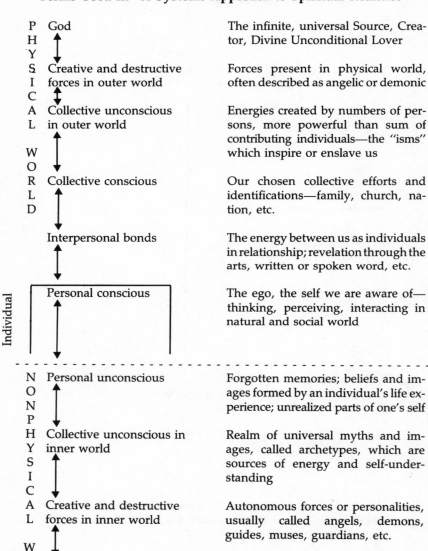

P H Y S I C A L W O R L D	**God**	The infinite, universal Source, Creator, Divine Unconditional Lover
	Creative and destructive forces in outer world	Forces present in physical world, often described as angelic or demonic
	Collective unconscious in outer world	Energies created by numbers of persons, more powerful than sum of contributing individuals—the "isms" which inspire or enslave us
	Collective conscious	Our chosen collective efforts and identifications—family, church, nation, etc.
	Interpersonal bonds	The energy between us as individuals in relationship; revelation through the arts, written or spoken word, etc.
Individual	**Personal conscious**	The ego, the self we are aware of—thinking, perceiving, interacting in natural and social world
N O N P H Y S I C A L W O R L D	**Personal unconscious**	Forgotten memories; beliefs and images formed by an individual's life experience; unrealized parts of one's self
	Collective unconscious in inner world	Realm of universal myths and images, called archetypes, which are sources of energy and self-understanding
	Creative and destructive forces in inner world	Autonomous forces or personalities, usually called angels, demons, guides, muses, guardians, etc.
	God	The infinite, universal Source, Creator, Divine Unconditional Lover

tween the individual, the unconscious, and the spiritual realm, we refer you to Morton Kelsey's outstanding book, *Psychology, Medicine and Christian Healing.*[16]

True healing is more than a cure of a specific complaint; it affects every dimension of the human person. Every healing system in the world, ancient and modern, secular and religious, has identified common elements of the healing process.[17]

First, there is the honest recognition of need: the person articulates his or her problem, accepts responsibility, and acknowledges his or her dependence on God for healing. Frequently, there is an invitation to encounter the Holy, which may come through a dream symbolically describing the problem.

Second, there is a pilgrimage or sacred journey to a consecrated place: a temple or healing shrine, a treatment center, hospital, support group, retreat center, or the sacred "inner space" of one's own interior.

Third, the person seeking healing goes through a ritual purification. Confession, personal inventory, ritual bathing, fasting, or other cleansing practices may be prescribed.

Fourth, altered states of consciousness are sought in order to allow contact with the unconscious, nonrational, nonmaterial spiritual realm. The expectation is that the unconscious holds the needed key to health, and willingly communicates it to us in a preverbal, symbolic language, if we will create the time and space to listen. The treasure we seek may come in the form of an infusion of new energy, insight, or change in the eidetic images that inform our belief system and impact our physical, emotional, and spiritual health (see chapter 2, "Emotional Dimension").

Generally, solitude and silence are sought in order to exclude external stimuli, so that the needed contents of the unconscious can cross over into conscious awareness and be noticed. Retreat, meditation, vision quest, rest, or forms of sensory deprivation may be used to allow the unconscious to become conscious. Sometimes consciousness is altered through communal rituals, and may include sensory stimulation, such as chanting, drumming, singing, and so on. Rituals of initiation, passage, healing, and celebration have power to change our perceptions of ourselves and of our relationships.

Altered states may occur spontaneously in the twilight states between waking and sleeping, daydreaming, listening to music, allowing one's mind to wander as we walk or run, becoming absorbed in work, reading, or art. Dangerous altered states can be induced through the use of drugs, for example, in which the conscious mind becomes overwhelmed. Safe, deliberately induced altered states can be produced by such techniques as guided imagery, meditation, chanting, and praying for healing dreams. A spiritual guide is essential to help sort out the symbolic contents of such reveries.

The difference between classical spiritual disciplines and other forms of altering one's state of consciousness is *intention*. For example, we may practice a form of psychological meditation, such as the relaxation response,[18] in order to reduce stress and to benefit one's physical and mental health. However, if it is our intention to deepen our relationship with God, we might meditate with a religious word or image, and our meditation becomes a prayer and a spiritual discipline. We can also be surprised by the spirit; for example, a recreational backpacking trip may become a life-transforming experience if one is overtaken by the Holy.

Opening up ourselves responsibly to the spiritual realm requires two important safeguards: first and most importantly, we must enter the spiritual dimension only in the name and spirit of God. Second, we must seek the guidance of an adviser, therapist, priest, or friend who is experienced with spiritual life.

We recognize that the unconscious, spiritual realm includes hostile as well as healing energies. To encounter the unconscious with absolute safety, one must do so under the protection of the Holy One, by whatever name we call upon God. We seek this divine protection by having the clear intention of growing in relationship with God, by imaging God's light surrounding us, by directly asking God to keep us safe from harm, or by approaching the unconscious through the avenue of sincere prayer.

We do not have the option of "playing it safe" by having nothing to do with the spiritual realm: the only alternative to meeting the spiritual dimension consciously is to meet it unconsciously, leaving ourselves open to influence by healing or hostile forces from within or from outside of us, without our awareness. The practice of spiritual disciplines with the intention of deepening relationship with God is the path of direct action, choice, and maximal physical, emotional, and spiritual health.

The authors recommend these classical spiritual disciplines: prayer, observing a Sabbath day, fasting, keeping a journal, and seeking spiritual guidance in order to achieve whole and holy living.

CLASSICAL SPIRITUAL DISCIPLINES

The term *classical spiritual disciplines* may conjure up images of monks chanting in an isolated monastery; however, spiritual disciplines are not just for vowed religious persons (or fanatics)—they are for everyone. For centuries, great spiritual teachers have practiced and taught religious practices that led to the experience of God. These practices, or spiritual disciplines, are central to the deeply felt knowledge and experience of God in our lives.[19]

The pace of modern life opposes our quest for God. Busy with deadlines, work, and full schedules, our lives are noisy with continual conversation, television and radio, even reading. Our senses are constantly bombarded, leaving no quiet spaces in which we might get in touch with our true Selves and with God. St. Augustine's words speak to us: "Our hearts will have no rest, until they rest in Thee, O Lord." That for which we yearn most of all is crowded out of our lives.

The classical spiritual disciplines create space. It is the space in our lives that gives our lives their definition, like the silence that surrounds and punctuates music, or the physical space which encompasses dance, or the relationship of positive and negative space in art. The light and the dark, the full and the empty, define each other. The space in our lives is fertile ground for creativity, just as the darkness of earth provides a womb for the seeds of new life.

The space created through the practice of spiritual disciplines may at first feel like emptiness. However, this emptiness can become a place of inner hospitality for God and for others, if that is our intention. Within it, we become attentive listeners, inviting God into ourselves and into our lives. Thus we allow God to become the center of our attention, rather than keeping our attention on ourselves. Spiritual disciplines enable us to become God-centered rather than self-centered, or egocentric. It is this shift in central focus that is the beginning of healing and change.

Change toward wholeness is God's work, not ours. We participate by making space for this work. The longer our journey toward wholeness, the more we realize that healing is not a personal accomplishment, but a gift of God. Our role is one of active consent and cooperation, in which we are open and attentive to God in our lives. This is how we allow ourselves to be changed by God's healing presence.

Being open to God means listening carefully and discerning which inner and outer voices are speaking God's word to us. God can come to us in our dreams, our everyday encounters with other people, through Scripture, through worship, through nature. God can also come to us through the daily newspaper, a phone call, through music, a word or a touch, an animal, a photograph. Even the most ordinary objects and occurrences of everyday life can be icons, or windows to the sacred. However, things are not always what they appear to be. Even the Evil One quotes Scripture for destructive purposes, as in the Gospel accounts of the temptation of Jesus. We have to know ourselves and our God well enough to recognize when God is reaching out to us.

The way to know ourselves and our God is through prayer. Prayer leads us into deeper union with God, so that what is holy in us recognizes the Holy whenever and wherever it may be found.

Sabbath, Solitude, and Silence

Sabbath, solitude, and silence create space in our lives to listen for the "still, small voice of God."[20] *Disciple*ship requires the *discipline* of attentive listening. Listening is at the heart of obedience, since it opens us to receive God's directive word, grace, and power in our lives.

Sabbath offers a foretaste of the reign of God, as a time of resting and rejoicing and remembering God's faithfulness and generosity. The Jewish people receive Sabbath as God's gift, "a rest granted in generous love, a true and faithful rest. . . . Let your children realize that their rest is from you, and by their rest may they sanctify your name."[21]

Truly, Sabbath exemplifies *kairos* time, the experience of the sacred within ordinary time. It is time set apart, consecrated, a sanctuary or cathedral in time. We would do well to follow the example of the Jewish observance of Sabbath, by consecrating time in our own lives to God alone. Resting, rejoicing, and remembering may be very difficult at first for busy, "productive" people, who feel that sacred rest is "wasting time." The practice of taking time to give ourselves to God alone often turns out to be a challenging discipline, as other interests and activities clamor for our time and attention.

Case Study

Joanne, a member of St. Luke Health Ministries' healing community, was very busy with the demands of raising young children several years ago when she began the practice of taking at least a half day each month to go to a nearby retreat center for a quiet time of prayer. Inevitably, when the arranged day would arrive, it would seem just the worst possible time to take a day off. The "worst" times to take a day for retreat are actually the best times to do it: she would return home relaxed and renewed, much better able to cope with the challenges and more efficient in getting things done. Spending time resting into awareness of God helped her to regain perspective on her relationship with God, to know herself better, and to receive the grace to continue giving herself to life and to others in a healthy way. Beginning to take Sabbath time was a significant turning point in her life, which led, one step at a time, into a deeper and richer spiritual life.

Solitude also helps us to get acquainted with ourselves. As we face our own strengths and weaknesses, our gentleness and compassion for others grow. We might fear solitude, confusing it with loneliness, but solitude is not lonely: God and our neighbors wait for us there. Entering into solitude, we find our true solidarity with others, our reverence for them, and our desire to respond to them grows strong. The paradox of solitude is that in going away from others, we actually deepen our ability to be with them.

Seeking solitude for healing seems instinctive. When we are sick, many of us seek seclusion in a quiet, undisturbed place in order to allow our bodies to heal. Similarly, healing of emotions, memories, mind, or spirit require making space for a certain "creative introversion," so that healing can come from within.[22]

Creativity frequently flows out of solitude. Composers, writers, artists, engineers, and inventors typically do much of their creative work in the crucible of solitude. Healthy, whole, and holy life is creative life, and it, too, requires solitude in order to stay in touch with the life-giving source within each of us. Solitude reorients us and transforms our lives.

One might ask— How can I find solitude in my busy household, my office or factory, my heavily populated life? Richard Foster encourages taking advantage of the "little solitudes" that might be found throughout an average day: during an early morning cup of coffee, standing in line, taking a bath, driving alone, or walking to the subway.[23]

Silence, like solitude, is a way of standing before God. Silence seems like risky business, because the truth of our humanity threatens to emerge and to be revealed *to us*. (God and our neighbors are already aware of our foibles.) These "dangerous" fresh perceptions deepen our sense of human frailty and giftedness, enabling us to become more compassionate.

Silence is more than simply not talking. It is listening to God within and around us. We give ourselves and our attention to God. The practice of avoiding speech for a period of time teaches us the deeper meaning of true silence, which is an inner quiet and attentiveness to God. Once we know what true silence feels like and how it works, we can begin to maintain inner quiet, even in the midst of activity and conversation.

Creating space within ourselves through Sabbath time and solitude, and cultivating inner silence eventually becomes habitual. This open space and inner quiet increases our desire to enter into dynamic relationship with God through prayer. Dynamic relationship means engaging in interaction with one another, and prayer is interacting with God who is available to be actively engaged with each of us.

Prayer and Meditation

Prayer is work—in fact, it is a joint effort: we extend ourselves by presenting ourselves and our needs to God, and God meets us and changes us.

Prayer is love in action—we express our longing for God by maintaining an awareness of God, a willingness to listen, an openness to change. God shows divine love for us by sharing God's own life with us, by forgiving us over and over again, and by leading us to wholeness.

Prayer is conversation between lovers—we speak to God about our lives, hopes, fears, feelings, needs; God speaks to us, words of comfort, encouragement, challenge, forgiveness, faith.

God's own spirit prays in us:[24] God initiates our prayer, prays in us, responds to us, heals us. God is not just the object of our prayer; God is the source. Prayer flows from the human spirit to God and back in an endless cycle, just as a stream flows out to the sea and is replenished by the rain.

Any thought, word, action, or feeling can become a prayer. Our intention transforms ordinary experience into prayer: if we seek to become aware of God's action in our lives, and if we are willing to listen and be changed, we are truly praying.

Richard Foster writes in *Celebration of Discipline*: "To pray is to change. Prayer is the central avenue God uses to transform us."[25] As God's own Spirit prays in us, we are transformed into the image of God:

Now this Lord is the Spirit, and where the Spirit of the Lord is, there is freedom. And we, with our unveiled faces reflecting like mirrors the brightness of the Lord, all grow brighter and brighter as we are turned into the image that we reflect; this is the work of the Lord who is Spirit.[26]

We encounter our Divine Lover through prayer, for God is infinitely available to us. Prayer often leads us into the inner wilderness . . . just as YHVH sought the conversion of God's nation in the book of Hosea: "I am going to lure her and lead her out into the wilderness and speak to her heart . . . There she will respond to me as she did when she was young. . . . "[27]

Psychologically speaking, prayer builds a relationship between the ego (the personal conscious) and the Self (the representation of God within).[28] As the Self becomes conscious and integrated, God is permitted to fill our lives from within, becoming an increasing source of identity and power. St. Paul beautifully articulates the experience of this transformation for the Christian in his prayer for the early church at Ephesus:

Out of his infinite glory, may [God] give you the power through his Spirit for *your hidden self to grow strong*, so that Christ may live in your hearts through faith, and then, planted in love and built on love, you will with all the saints have strength to grasp the breadth and the length, the height and the depth; until, knowing the love of Christ, which is beyond all knowledge, *you are filled with the utter fullness of God.*[29] [authors' italics]

Prayer does not require fancy words or formal structures; nor do we need special titles or training to speak to God. All we need to do is be ourselves and pray from the heart. The Psalms offer an excellent example of heartfelt prayers poured out in plain, direct words addressed to God in a very familiar way.

Each person can develop a prayer style that suits his or her personality and life-style. The important thing is to pray. Praise God. Give thanks. Ask for specific blessings for yourself or for loved ones. Sing. Dance. Seek forgiveness. Pray alone. Pray with others. Pray for healing.

There are as many ways to pray, and as many reasons to pray, as there are people. One may take a morning cup of coffee to a quiet place to spend that time with God. Another might pray with the newspaper, asking God's grace to enter the many situations that cry out for justice and healing. Still another may pray while walking or jogging. Some may send short prayers, what St. Theresa called "heavenward glances," all through the day. Some people pray with Scriptures, studying and then reflecting on a passage, perhaps carrying a meaningful word or verse in their hearts all day long. Many find communal prayer meaningful: worshiping with a church community, participating in services of healing, praying with family in the home. Or a person may feel drawn to one of the many forms of meditation that lend themselves so well to listening as well as speaking to God.

Meditation is an altered state of consciousness characterized by concentrated attention. This occurs spontaneously when we become pleasantly absorbed in what we are doing, who we are with, or the beauty of a place. We are also capable of learning to meditate so that we can enter a relaxed, alert state at will. Meditation offers many physical, psychological, and spiritual benefits, including stress management, deep relaxation, getting in touch with feelings or images, tapping creativity, or inviting the Holy into our lives. Meditation may be primarily "secular" and psychological or it can be profoundly religious. If one's primary purpose is to focus attention on God, desiring to deepen relationship with God, then meditation becomes prayer. Meditation as prayer might focus on a religious word, passage, story, or imagery from an individual's faith tradition, or it might consist of a highly disciplined openness to God who is beyond all of our words and images, in a form of contemplative prayer.

Much of our prayer consists of talking to God, or talking *at* God. Listening is essential to true conversation with God. Prayerful meditation offers a way to *listen* for "the still, small voice of God." There are many forms of meditation; two that we recommend highly are meditating with Scripture and centering prayer.

Meditation begins with finding a suitable place, free from interruptions. You may need to turn off the telephone and retreat to a quiet room, or at least out of the mainstream of activity in your home or workplace. Meditation outdoors can be wonderful, with the heat, rain, cool breezes, the beauty and power of nature, songs of birds, the color of the sky, the dampness of the ground—whatever the conditions, elements of nature often turn our attention to the Creator. The sounds of the city can also be allowed into meditation, if one meditates in an office, with phones ringing, typewriters and computers printing, human voices, and the sounds of city traffic simply allowed to be the background.

Find a comfortable position, but not so comfortable that you fall asleep as soon as you relax. Most people find that keeping their backs straight is the least fatiguing position to hold for a period of meditation. This might be accomplished sitting cross-legged on the floor, or on a cushion or prayer bench made especially for meditation, or by sitting in a straight-backed chair with both feet flat on the ground. Some people (who are not too tired) meditate comfortably lying flat on the floor, feet slightly apart, palms up, pelvis tilted so the curve of the back rests on the floor in a stressless position. The object is to find a posture that you can comfortably maintain without fatigue or pain for a chosen period of time, and which gives you the freedom to focus your concentration inward, rather than paying constant attention to your body as you meditate. You want your body relaxed and your mind alert.

The next step involves getting in touch with your intention to give your entire self to God. This time is consecrated and undivided—you choose not to do anything else right now except to be with God. Ask for the help you need to be truly willing to give yourself completely to prayer, or tell God in your own words of your longing for deeper relationship. Know that God loves you and waits for you. God is our safe shelter as we enter the unexplored regions of the unconscious: "I sing for joy in the shadow of your wings; my soul clings close to you, your right hand supports me."[30]

Let go of the tensions, busy-ness, and preoccupations of the day, by closing your eyes to focus inward, or by using a simple object such as a lighted candle or icon or any meaningful symbol for you as a focal point. Take three or four *slow*, deep breaths, imagining yourself inhaling peacefulness and exhaling tension. At this point, you are ready to move into meditation with Scripture or centering prayer.

To meditate with Scripture, you might choose to enter into a selected Scripture story imaginatively, filling in the sensory details of the setting, then reflecting on how the event must have appeared and felt to various characters in the story. Or perhaps you might choose a word, a phrase, a verse, or an image from the passage, and spend some time with that, repeating it over and over quietly in your mind in rhythm with your breathing. This method of praying with Scripture allows the living word of God to take root gradually in your heart.

To practice centering prayer, allow yourself to rest into the presence of God dwelling deep within you. Perhaps a single word will come to you to express the quality of God's love and presence that you experience. Some of the words individuals have shared with us include the name "Jesus," or "Yeshua," the words "Abba," "Shalom," "Father," "Mother," "Grandmother," "echad," "peace," "mercy," or any of the titles or names for God that are meaningful to us.

Whenever distracting thoughts float through our awareness, we can notice them and let them flow by, returning gently to the word that keeps us centered in God's presence. Spend several minutes, perhaps 10 to 15 minutes at first, increasing gradually to 30 minutes or even an hour. The length of time we spend in meditation is pretty irrelevant, except as a sign of our love and commitment to God. God can do great things in whatever space we allow.

At the end of your meditation time, a gentle transition may be made by mentally praying a formal prayer, such as the "Our Father," or a little prayer in your own words of thanksgiving and praise. Begin to stretch and move your body slowly, open your eyes, and very gently resume normal activities.

Meditation does not have to be motionless—we can meditatively interpret a Scripture story through dance, or practice centering prayer while walking or running. People sometimes practice centering prayer while doing absorbing, but safe, repetitive work, such as knitting, weaving, crafts, housework, or gardening.

Another form of meditation that lends itself to knowing God and ourselves better consists of fully bringing our attention to the present moment. Since we believe that God is in everything and everyone, there lies an opportunity in every moment to meet God: in folding clothes, changing the oil in the car, preparing food, making love, listening to a neighbor, caring for a sick child, attending a meeting, paying the bills. So many people say they do not have time for a spiritual life, especially single parents struggling to make ends meet financially and to take care of the endless needs of their children. God is infinitely available in the moment; our task is to maintain a willingness to see, to be touched, and to be changed by the Holy in the everyday stuff of life. Raising a child and paying the bills can be a spiritual discipline, and it can be a meditation, if we open ourselves to that possibility.

Focusing our attention on the present moment is both extraordinarily simple and extraordinarily difficult. The challenge lies in acknowledging and embracing *all* of life. Buddhist monk and Zen master Thich Nhat Hanh describes meditation in this manner:

> Meditation is to be aware of what is going on—in our bodies, in our feelings, in our minds, and in the world. Each day 40,000 children die of hunger. The superpowers now have more than 50,000 nuclear warheads, enough to destroy our planet many times. Yet the sunrise is beautiful, and the rose that bloomed this morning along the wall is a

miracle. Life is both dreadful and wonderful. To practice meditation is
to be in touch with both aspects.[31]

Christians who want to know more about prayer are referred to
With Open Hands, by Henri Nouwen; much valuable help and practical
suggestions on meditation can be found in *Centering Prayer*, by
M. Basil Pennington, and *The Journey Toward Wholeness*, by Kenneth
Bakken and Kathleen Hofeller. Those who feel drawn to prayerful
meditation rooted in the Buddhist tradition will find a wealth of insight in *A Gradual Awakening*, by Stephen Levine, and *Being Peace*, by
Thich Nhat Hanh. Meditation in the Jewish tradition is beautifully
explained in *Jewish Meditation*, by Aryeh Kaplan. Those who prefer
to begin with "secular" meditation for emotional and physical health
can get started with *The Relaxation Response*, by Herbert Benson, and
Minding the Body, Mending the Mind, by Joan Borysenko.[32]

Just as the time we give to God signals our commitment, so does
paying attention to what we experience in our prayer time and the
whole of our inner and outer journeys. Fresh insights are often very
fragile and surprisingly fleeting. One moment's astounding "aha!"
all too soon becomes an irretrievable memory unless it is written down
right away. The insights along our healing journeys must be recorded
in order to become integrated into our lives. The backs of envelopes
and sticky notepapers are only temporary aids to memory until the
event or insight can be placed in a more permanent record.

Keeping a Journal

Keeping a journal provides a valuable container for the contents of our
prayer, meditations, dreams, experiences, moods, fantasies, and feelings. We need to treasure all of this raw material in order for its
healing potential to become realized in our lives. Many thoughts,
feelings, and experiences seem "charged" with an unusually strong
response in us at the time when they occur, alerting us to the need
to pay attention. Recording the events of our spiritual journeys in a
safe place demonstrates that we value them and are willing to attend
to them.

A journal can be a record of God's faithfulness to us and an invitation for us to be faithful in response. We have seen that God communicates with us through the unconscious. Morton Kelsey describes

the journal as a collection of love letters from God, and states that the act of writing them down keeps them coming.[33]

The journal is a remarkable tool. It gives us a little distance from ourselves, so that we can look at ourselves more objectively. It strengthens the ego, so that we are not overwhelmed by the unconscious. It allows our unconscious minds to work for us—solving problems, thinking creatively, making decisions, understanding another person's point of view, conversing with different parts of ourselves.

We might think that anything this helpful must be difficult, expensive, and must certainly require some kind of expertise. In fact, it is probably the least expensive, most helpful, simplest, self-care tool available. All that is required is a bound book—a simple spiral notebook does just fine—and a pen or pencil. It is not necessary to be able to write or spell well. A willingness to be honest, to play with ideas and words, and to be open to possibilities is all that is needed.

Privacy and the freedom to express anything and everything in an honest, nonjudgmental manner are key elements to creating a journal that can truly help us toward wholeness. The dark, violent, hateful, or helpless aspects of our inner life are usually *just as precious* as the light, compassionate, loving, and strong parts of ourselves. All of the images and feelings of the inner life need to be brought into the light of our awareness, into our journal, and hopefully, into our prayer, in order for us to become healed, whole, and holy. We may misunderstand the "negative" feelings and images ourselves; we must thus protect ourselves and others from the unnecessary pain or misunderstanding that could come from leaving our journals where someone else may read them.

What goes into a journal? What you *don't* want is a running account of daily events. Instead, record ideas—planting them like seeds in your journal so they can develop in your unconscious mind, with almost no effort on the part of your conscious mind. Later, these inspirations return in an expanded form, to be replanted in your journal so they can continue to grow.[34] It is helpful to record events or encounters that you sense intuitively as having significance which invites exploration. Notes, quotes, dreams, reflections, prayers, drawings, feelings, fantasies, questions, struggles, hopes, fears, imaginative dialogues with parts of ourselves, or with persons living or dead, decision-making processes—all these and more can be stored in the treasure chest of a personal journal.

A journal for the care of the whole person would include notes on physical preventive health care as well as jottings from the emotional and spiritual life. The journal might include notes about foods consumed, relating eating patterns to mood, activity, relationships, alertness, or energy level. It can be a place to keep track of progress with your exercise program, to observe changes in how you feel physically, to watch whether or not you are keeping your life in balance, keeping your stress level down, getting enough sleep, rest, and recreation.

For many, the most important use of a journal is for *dreamwork*, recording dreams and exploring their meaning. God can speak to us through our unconscious through dreams, and Scriptures offer many history-changing examples. Our own life histories can be changed toward health through the symbolic language of dreams.

Some dreams have more to do with the unfinished business of the day than they do with divine revelation. Paying attention to dreams enables us to distinguish significant dreams from those that are insignificant. Elaine and a friend "catch up" periodically by telling each other a recent dream, without interpretation. In minutes, they are in touch with each other at a level that would otherwise take hours or days of conversation. It is not mysterious; we learn the language of the unconscious the way we learn our native language—by listening, paying attention, and beginning to use it. The journal offers an excellent way to listen, pay attention, increase our skill, and put the insight we gain to work for us.

Pray for dreams that will give insight into your life situation. Record the dream, the parts you remember, and any feelings about it, as soon as possible. Some people find it helpful to keep a notepad and pen or pencil, or a tape recorder beside their beds. Enter into the dream by recording it in the first person, present tense. For example, "I am in a clearing in the woods, several people are standing in small groups . . . ." Later, you may dialogue imaginatively with different parts of the dream, knowing that each part of the dream is some aspect of yourself. You can pray with it or about it; explore it by painting or drawing or dancing it; talk about it with others who understand dreams and work with them; complete a dream or change the ending if you wish; and pray for additional dreams if the meaning remains unclear.

For more suggestions about healing, creative journal-keeping, and dreamwork, we refer you to *The New Diary*, by Tristine Rainer, and *Adventure Inward*, by Morton Kelsey. Both books open up exciting possibilities for the beginning and the seasoned journal writer, and both contain chapters on dreamwork. Rainer's book is for readers of any faith tradition or no faith tradition; Kelsey's is written from the Christian perspective, as is *Dreams and Spiritual Growth*, by Savary, Berne, and Williams—an outstanding source on dreamwork.[35]

*   *   *

Spiritual disciplines, particularly prayer and meditation, bring us face
to face with Mystery—the mystery of ourselves; the inner life, eternal
life; and the Source of all life. Mystery evokes an intense magnetic
attraction as our whole nature responds with joyful recognition. We
also respond with awe and trembling before the Infinite. Words,
images, and comprehension become inadequate. Old beliefs, perceptions, patterns of behavior, images of ourselves, and images of God
have to change. Suddenly, or gradually, we are suspended between
our fixed, secure notions of reality and the unknown. The only thing
to do is also the most terrifying: *surrender* the familiar and reach for
the unknown.

Changing behavior by letting go of limiting beliefs is difficult and
frightening. It requires the reassurance, encouragement, and guidance of others who have walked this way before. We need someone
who knows that breaking out of old patterns and yielding to Infinite
Love is precisely the point where God touches our lives and we are
healed.

So, this is healing! No wonder we fear healing as desperately as
we want it. It feels like dying, and indeed, it is dying to our old selves.
How can we be sure that dying to the old is being born to the new?
How can we let go of the known and secure, and reach for the unknown, unlimited possibility? We would have to be crazy or else have
tremendous faith. Or perhaps, we could make the leap based on the
faith of people with whom we have trusting relationships.

Guidance

Guidance is the discipline of seeking relationship with others who can
help us. We have to identify our needs carefully in order to seek
appropriate helpers and companions. We may need to seek a physician, a faith community, a psychotherapist, a spiritual guide or
friend, or all of these.

A physician with an appreciation of the body/mind/spirit relationship can be helpful both in prevention and treatment of disease.
Ideally, this person would encourage active agency on the part of the
"patient," or health-care participant, and would be open to complementary healing modalities. As Bernie Siegel points out, "Patients
who want to get well through the doctor alone or God alone are
minimizing their chances." Siegel sees his role as physician as "not
only to find the right treatment but to help the patient find an inner
reason for living, resolve conflicts, and free healing energy."[36] Good

medical treatment gives the person freedom from symptoms, so one can have the best chance to find lasting, inner healing. Good medical care both manages the disease and attends the process of finding meaning in one's experience of sickness and health. This can be done by a gifted physician alone or through the collaboration of a health-care providing team.

A faith tradition offers roots and a guiding light for our journeys. Meaning can be found through connecting our personal stories with a larger story. For example, a Christian who is in touch with his or her own experience can identify with a moment in the life of Jesus. Such an identification places the particular event in our own lives within a significant context, enabling us to remain anchored in faith rather than helplessly adrift in life's inevitable stormy periods. We will have heard the rest of the story. Those who feel they are wandering in a desert period in their lives know that God's people were led into the promised land. Those who suffer as Jesus did in the garden of Gethsemane or in his Crucifixion know that death does not have the final word.

A faith community can be a source of guidance and encouragement, as well as an opportunity to encounter God. Communal worship, faith sharing, rituals, sacraments, and hearing the word of God read and preached all offer us the opportunity to approach God and to allow God the opportunity to touch our lives. A worshiping community can be a living reminder of God's faithfulness, since God has been a part of its corporate history and its members' personal histories over time. The community or its individual members can remind one another that God is with each of them. Communities that attempt to listen carefully to the leading of God's Spirit can offer assistance in discerning God's will for their members.

Many persons have had profound experiences of God's grace through the process of psychotherapy. This may be offered by "secular" professionals such as psychiatrists, psychologists, social workers, or other mental health professionals, or by religious professionals such as pastoral counselors, or ministers or chaplains with psychological training. The provider may be secular or religious—the language may be different, but the potential for healing is the same. Anyone who is seeking a therapist can pray for guidance, ask for recommendations from trusted friends, interview several therapists, and *trust one's own intuitions*. Caring, commitment, discipline, knowledge, and humility are essential qualities for a good therapist. Psychotherapy is an intense, intimate relationship; it is worth making the effort at the very beginning to find the right therapist.

Some therapists deal directly with religious and spiritual issues; others leave the work of integrating therapy with one's own faith to the client; some therapists believe religious conviction is a sign of pathology. Any person seeking personal and spiritual growth through therapy needs to know where the therapist stands.

Classical spiritual guidance or spiritual friendship is a disciplined, intimate relationship for the purpose of attending to God's grace at work in one person's life. Ordinarily a person seeking spiritual guidance is motivated by a desire to deepen relationship with God. The person who acts as a spiritual guide for others must be committed to his or her own spiritual journey and be familiar with the dynamics of relationship with God—including desire, resistance, discernment, surrender, attachment, willfulness, forgiveness, awareness, and true humility—as well as an understanding of spiritual disciplines. The meetings focus on God's presence and activity in an individual's life, experiences of prayer, and how God invites the person to grow in any part of his or her life—relationships, vocation, social justice, sexuality, priorities, to name a few possibilities. God's own Spirit is recognized as the true director in a spiritual direction relationship.

Sometimes a person in emotional pain seeks spiritual guidance. The spiritual guide may believe that a referral to a psychotherapist is necessary instead of, or in addition to, being in spiritual guidance. These disciplines are complementary and may be offered by one individual trained in both, or by members of an interdisciplinary team.

Fasting as a spiritual discipline is abstaining, usually from food, for the purpose of glorifying God. A fast may be partial, abstaining from certain foods, or total, abstaining from all solid or liquid food except water. Food often pacifies uncomfortable feelings inside us; fasting presents us with an opportunity to discover what in us cries out for healing. Fasting also shows us the intensity of our attachment to food or to anything else in our lives that could enslave us. There are many secondary benefits of the spiritual discipline of fasting: clarity of mind, health of body, weight loss, growth in self-discipline. We say more about the benefits of fasting, and give suggestions on how to fast, in chapter 5.

Spiritual disciplines enable us to experience God in a personal way, enhance self-knowledge, and deepen our awareness of the interconnectedness of all persons and all creation. They are ways that we can demonstrate our commitment to God and to our own healing process. Spiritual disciplines can create balance, space, and rhythm in our lives that enhance physical, emotional, spiritual, and social well-being.

Time and effort invested in spiritual practices open us to the experience of the sacred within the commonplace. The careful management of our time becomes critically important in developing a lifestyle with room for the spiritual dimension. The investment of time is richly rewarded with the transformation of our experience of time, from ordinary busy-ness to extraordinary grace.

The point of any spiritual discipline is the removal of barriers to the experience of God. Most barriers are based on prevalent illusions and attitudes toward life. By attending to these fundamental issues, we can be more open to God, experience freedom from unnecessary suffering and stress, and consequently live healthier, happier lives. We turn our attention now to 10 core issues, which we develop into positive principles for healthy, holy living.

4

A Prescription for Abundant Life

Our approach to life may be compared to how we might approach a river. We may choose to swim downstream, sometimes resting and allowing the river to carry us along. We may decide to swim across the current to the other side, or we may attempt to swim upstream against the flow. Another possibility might be to get into a boat and not make contact with the water at all. We may then navigate the water from the safety of the boat either downstream, upstream, or across the current.

Life is like flowing water, sometimes gentle, sometimes overpowering. We are always in relationship with it. We have choices about how we want to relate to life: moving with it, working against it, being carried by it, or trying to stay a safe distance from it.

To enter into life fully is to experience God. Health, healing, and holiness mean being in open exchange with God and life. Abundant life means risking being open to all of it—the joy and the pain, the loves and the losses. The moment we begin to be selective about what we are willing to experience, we put limitations on our experience of God and life. Often we resist painful realities because we believe that life is not supposed to be this way. We are called to enter into life the way it is: sometimes hard, sometimes joyful, always beyond our full comprehension.

At the heart of any spiritual discipline is the desire to remove barriers to our relationship with God. Examples of common barriers include: allowing our lives to get off-center, holding onto control, denial, worrying about the future, feeling guilt about the past, dualistic thinking, denying one's Self, clinging to emotional or intellectual security, craving, addictions, rationalizing, preoccupation, and avoidance. The classical spiritual disciplines heighten our awareness of these deeper issues. From these fundamental issues we can develop positive principles which enhance an open exchange with God, life, and our social, spiritual, and natural world.

Regardless of our state of health, or age, or the challenges we may face, these disciplines enable us to reduce unnecessary suffering and stress, and to live more fully and freely. The following 10 disciplines are a prescription for whole, holy, healthy living.

Keep God at the Center

Single-mindedness and single-heartedness are rare among human beings. More typical is a kind of unreflected life, one in which we make choices and act, unaware of our motivations and compulsions. Our energies may be dissipated among many competing interests and desires, or they may be focused around something important to us. Evelyn Underhill observed that people generally center whole sections of their lives around "ambition, love, duty, friendship, social convention, politics, religion, self-interest in one of its myriad forms," only to find that each of these must eventually fail them or enslave them.[1]

We might even drift unaware into creating several centers in our lives simultaneously, finding our hearts and minds "full of little whirlpools, twists and currents, conflicting systems, incompatible desires."[2] Even the most positive values, such as those listed by Underhill, or family, ministry, or work are as potentially idolatrous as the recognizably destructive ones, such as centering a life around money, sex, alcohol, power, materialism, or disease. *Anything* can creep into a central position in our lives if we are not attentive, causing us to compromise our faithfulness to God's will.

By arranging everything we hold dear in life around one center, God alone, life becomes simpler and more free-flowing. We are then able to listen for the will of God as it applies to every part of our lives. The energies once caught up into whirlpools within are freed for love, obedience to God, self-discipline, and self-giving.

We need to be attentive to the following questions:

What is *most* important to me? What do I plan my life around? Do I have one center, or several?

How do I experience my energies—as focused, dissipated, absent, compulsive, fragmented, or free-flowing?

Where does God fit into my life?

Do I sometimes feel the need to try to "be God" by trying to be a savior of sorts?

Trust the Process

If we trust God to be God, then we don't have to try to be God. We stop wrestling control over life from God, and enjoy the freedom of being responsible just for ourselves. This freedom is built on trust: God is trustworthy.

Our experiences have taught us fear, so our tendency is to cling to whatever control we imagine possible. Henri Nouwen, in his book on prayer, *With Open Hands*, tells the story of an old woman who was brought into a psychiatric ward. She clenched a single coin in a tight fist, swinging and fighting as though her very life depended on hanging onto that coin.[3] Like her, we cling to our fears, beliefs, disappointments, anger, meanness, as though our lives depend on them; indeed, our secure, limited self-knowledge does depend on them. This clinging uses up much of our energy: willfulness is stressful. We may want to let go and open our hands to God and to each other in receptivity, but we seem unable to do it.

How can we relax into peaceful surrender to God's love? We can begin by noticing where we are in relationship to divine love and pray from there. Perhaps most of us will need to pray for the grace to let go of control, and for supportive, encouraging companions and teachers, and for experiences of love that will heal the experiences which taught fear. YHVH offers the coin of compassion, waiting patiently and lovingly for us to be able to reach out in open acceptance.

We need to ask ourselves:

Where in my life am I trying to *make* something happen? What do I fear will happen if I do not take control of the situation?

As I reflect on a particular situation, do I feel open to the *full range* of possibilities, or do I feel willful about how I want things to be?

Live in the Present

There is no such thing as a dull moment. Every moment is an opportunity for abundant life, if we are willing to open to the encounter of the extraordinary in the ordinary. The Holy and the Infinite are met in doing what we are doing—attentively. Often our perceptions are clouded by fears of the past and anxieties about the future, rather than being open to the present moment, with our senses alert, our hearts and minds receptive, our being grounded in hopeful expectation.

The present moment holds the peace we seek. We need only enter the experience fully, whatever it may be. It may contain joy, service to others, caring for ourselves, suffering, loss, connecting: the full range of human experience can be a window into Divine Mystery.

Some of our past experiences have taught us to fear, causing us to erect walls around our hearts. This inner barricade once protected us from abandonment or pain. Unfortunately, it also limits our capacity to give and receive love. Joan Borysenko writes that "to go on protecting ourselves once the situation has passed and, worse, to see the old situation where it does not exist are equivalent to building a prison and then volunteering to live in it."[4] Healing involves stepping out of bondage, invited and empowered by grace.

Anxiety about the future, fantasizing a future as an escape from the present, or wanting something (setting up conditions for happiness), are all at the root of a lot of unnecessary suffering. Perhaps one waits impatiently for a bus, thus missing the opportunity to enjoy people-watching, the color of the sky, or the moment of solitude. Or maybe one's situation is as difficult as living with an alcoholic family member. In this case, a spiritually based 12-step program, Al-Anon, has shown countless people how to reduce their suffering by simultaneously facing the reality of the present moment and letting go of the desire for things to be different in order to be happy. This path of letting go of wishing sets an example for us all. The "Serenity Prayer" contains wisdom we can live by: "God grant me the serenity to accept the things I cannot change; the courage to change the things I can; and the wisdom to know the difference."

Living in the present moment, being mindful of what is and what we are doing now, is simplicity itself, but it is not easy. For example, if we are folding clothes, taking a shower, or talking to a child, our minds may wander away unless we teach them to stay attentive. If the situation is really difficult: caring for someone we love who is dying, living with a lifeless marriage, or feeling stuck in a dead-end job, mindful attention to the present becomes that much harder. Looking away from the present is the essence of "living in neutral." If we want to be on the path toward healing and wholeness, we must begin by faithfully paying attention to the present situation.

We are called to reflect:

How are my thoughts, feelings, or actions governed by fears from the past or desires for the future?

What might I be avoiding by turning my attention away from the present situation? Boredom? Lack of freedom? Intimacy? Truth? A need for change?

Be Attuned to What Is

Opening ourselves to the present moment places us face to face with reality. The truth does indeed set us free, but not without "paying our dues." The cost of that freedom is letting go of judgments, and of the security of preconceived ideas, illusions, rationalizations, and denial. We also have to stop projecting undesirable aspects of ourselves onto others. Standing between freedom at such a cost and unfreedom with its attractive security usually feels like being caught between a rock and a hard place: choosing truth requires enormous courage.

It helps to let go of the need to judge everything and everyone, including ourselves. Joan Borysenko describes different aspects of the mind in helpful terms, attributing the judging attribute to the ego, the open witnessing attribute to the true Self. The ego is conditioned by our personal life experiences and seeks the security of dividing everything into neat categories of good or bad, black and white; the Self is not conditioned by personal experience and so the Self accepts how things are.[5] The true Self observes with total compassion, enabling us to see the truth, to "tell it like it is," and to be set free.

Living the truth requires great humility, that is, knowing ourselves, and being ourselves. We have to own our strengths and weaknesses, the beautiful and the broken parts of ourselves, the light and the dark, the reality of who we are now, and also the wonder of our originally blessed nature. This honest self-acceptance leads to compassion for ourselves and for others. It also means that we have no need to hide the truth of who we are from ourselves or anyone else.

Our task is to see the world around us, our work and our relationships clearly, and to name accurately that which promotes life and wholeness, and that which brings destruction and death, from small, subtle matters to issues on the global scale. Courage is essential to face the truth in life, rather than settle for illusion, rationalization, denial, or any of the ways available to us to protect us from any reality that is painful to us.

Our feelings are often the vehicle for discovering what is true in our situations, relationships, interactions, and thoughts. Getting in touch with what is depends very much on attentiveness to what we actually feel. A nonjudgmental, accepting attitude is needed in relation to our feelings. There are no unacceptable feelings: our feelings are okay; acting them out may be another story. Feelings themselves are an appropriate, automatic, physiological, and emotional response. If we refuse to acknowledge our feelings, they remain hidden from our awareness and surface unexpectedly some other time, demanding to be heard. The best policy is to allow our feelings as they arise, neither resisting them nor clinging to them. Then they can work for us, calling our attention to the truth of what is happening, enabling us to choose consciously how to respond.

Authenticity, the hallmark of whole and holy living, means living in such a way that who we are, what we believe, what we do, how we relate to others and to nature, and the flowing life of the universe are in harmony. This requires constant growth in awareness of what is true about ourselves, our natural, technological, and spiritual world, our relationships, our God. And it requires great humility to face ourselves honestly, owning our strengths and weaknesses, our compassion and our violence, our generosity and our rigidity, our love and our fear.

Living the truth sets us free from all pretense and fear, when we no longer need our defensive barriers, illusions, or anything our minds once needed to protect us. The energy once used for defending one's illusions becomes free to use in more creative, life-giving ways. Also, with the removal of barriers between ourselves and God's Spirit, the divine life of God can flow into and through us as the source of genuine empowerment.

Freedom demands Self-giving. The energies previously engaged in protecting us from the truth, once liberated, need to become a gift. The unique incarnation of God's love that we are demands expression. It is not only our own energy that becomes available, but as barriers are removed within us, we become more open channels for God's own Spirit to flow through us into our world. Spiritual life is shared life; spirit longs for union with God's Spirit everywhere, in everyone.

In order to be attuned to what is, we need to ask ourselves:

What is it that I do not want to see about my life, my self, my situation? How can I let in this awareness—first, without judgment, and then, allowing it to be surrounded with merciful forgiveness and kindness?

What do I love or hate in others, that perhaps I do not see in myself?

What am I feeling in a given situation? Why? How does this affect me physically? How does it affect me socially—does it draw me toward others in love, or into withdrawn isolation?

What next step would lead me toward increased awareness, freedom, acceptance, forgiveness, connection, mercy, and compassion?

Live Creatively with Paradox

When we pay attention to our feelings, and honestly face how things are, we often find that apparent opposites are frequently true at the same time. Life is full of paradox: there is loss in winning; there is peace in suffering; there is death in birth, and birth in death. Making sense of life by dividing everything into "either/or" categories does not work for long. When we fully enter into our experience, we begin to see that "both/and" thinking corresponds more closely with reality.

Dualistic thinking is a Eurocentric idea rooted in Hellenistic philosophy, expanded and overlaid with (mis)interpretations of Christianity. The Hebrew, African, Eastern, and native American cultures have consistently held a more integrated understanding of how "opposites" are intertwined. In these religious and cultural belief systems, body and spirit, creativity and destructiveness, divinity and nature are inseparable. Regardless of our individual backgrounds within the cultural melting pot of the United States, our institutions have largely been informed and dominated by European, quasi-Christian dualism. (Western Christians will find much healing of this dualistic thinking by recalling the Jewishness of Jesus that runs through his teachings and living example, and by acquainting themselves with Christian creation-centered spirituality.)[6]

Some of the either/or pairs we can do without include:

good/bad	black/white
happiness/suffering	sick/healthy
male/female	win/lose
birth/death	body/spirit
divinity/humanity	creative/destructive

Joseph Campbell describes the Garden of Eden as "the place of unity, of nonduality of male and female, good and evil, God and human beings."[7] Eating the fruit of duality, the tree of knowledge of good and evil, is choosing to leave the Garden; discovering that God and self and others and creation are one is choosing to return to the Garden.

The experience of dualistic perception is a kind of Crucifixion, with contradictory, irreconcilable opposites pulling us apart inside. Eastern philosophy, on the other hand, recognizes opposing energies that need to be in balance for life to be harmonious. If we can tolerate the tension of opposites existing within each other, rather than tearing us apart, the experience of paradox will lead us toward Mystery, an awe-filled recognition of the Holy.

In order to locate where we may be thinking dualistically, we can ask ourselves:

Where do I find myself torn between options in my life, whether in perceptions, thinking, or concrete situations? Do I really need to choose between opposites, or is there a way for both options to be workable and true at the same time?

Is there room in me for "both/and" thinking? Might I experience peace in suffering, awe in tragedy, strength in surrender?

Am I able to take in new perceptions of myself and my world and integrate them without throwing out everything I ever knew about myself before?

Can I see myself as saint and sinner, strong and vulnerable, peaceful and aggressive, loving and fearful, faithful and wandering, a healer and a person in need of healing?

Forgive

Recognizing the opposites within ourselves often places us in a position of needing to forgive ourselves. Opening ourselves to experience life as it is may create the need to forgive others, and sometimes even to forgive God.

Being in touch with our feelings means that sometimes we will feel hurt, betrayed, abandoned, angry, discouraged, or depressed. These appropriate, automatic feelings call our attention to an injustice that needs our response; however, our natural instinct is to retreat into emotional isolation in an attempt to protect ourselves from additional hurt, or to retaliate. Unfortunately, this instinctive, but guarded, position is a major block to healing. Now what? Jesus answered with the most unexpected, unnatural, unlikely, unimaginable response: "Love your enemies and pray for those who persecute you" (Matt. 5:44). The astounding truth is that forgiveness is the active choice for the freedom, health, and wholeness *of the forgiver*!

Forgiveness is often misunderstood. It sometimes appears to be a shortcut, leaping to understanding and acceptance without dealing with the reality of the wound, the hurt, and the anger. Or it may appear to be an expression of passivity, helplessness, resignation, or victimization. None of these imposters for forgiveness does justice to the real courage, choice, and active agency that characterize authentic forgiveness.

Forgiveness is a process that begins where we are, and it cannot be rushed without emotional violence to ourselves. Perhaps the place we typically begin is with being in touch with the pain of injury, wanting the wounding to stop, and wanting to be able to forgive. We can pray through our feelings for the grace to grow into forgiveness. That respect for ourselves, honoring the integrity and timing of the forgiveness process, allows change to take place. We still have to deal with the injury and take steps to stop it from continuing. Gradually we begin to see ourselves and the one who has hurt us in a different light. We become empowered to go beyond the pain, and from a position of strength, we can refuse to be programmed by those who have hurt us. Thus the cycle of retaliation is broken, and new life is possible.

Many people find it easier to forgive others than to forgive themselves. Forgiving ourselves is a necessary prerequisite to being able to receive others' forgiveness, including God's. This means accepting ourselves without judgment, allowing ourselves to be "only" human and fully human—persons with strengths and weaknesses and with the dignity of God's children. God's love is unconditional, like the love of a grandparent who delights in the antics, exuberance, clumsiness, curiosity, and messiness of a young grandchild. God already loves, forgives, and accepts us—can we let go of our judgments in order to let God's love in?

We sometimes feel that God is responsible for our suffering. Amid life's hurts, we may find ourselves being angry with God, consciously or unconsciously. God is big enough to hear our angry, tearful tirades. Then we need to be quiet in order to hear God's response within us. All of the world's religions struggle with the problem of human suffering. There are no easy answers, or surely they would have been found by now. There is comfort in allowing God to be with us in our pain.

God is with us—that unbearable mystery is at the heart of the (often troublesome) story of the Crucifixion of Jesus: that he opened his arms on the cross in the most generous act of union with all human suffering, carrying out his unique, sacrificial vocation of atonement (at-one-ment). Jesus then practiced what he preached—with full awareness of the pain and injustice he suffered, with fidelity to his vocation of union with all human suffering throughout all time, with authenticity and active choice, he set himself and his persecutors free: "Father, forgive them; they do not know what they are doing."[8]

When we can name the wound, feel the pain, be angry about the injustice, do what we can to stop the injustice from continuing, and choose to forgive—*that* is choosing freedom and life. When we allow ourselves to be channels of God's mercy so that unconditional love can enter into a hurtful situation—*that* is healing. Forgiveness is not instinctive and it is not easy; it requires that we rise above ourselves, going beyond conditioned responses, in order to be free. One who can truly forgive has accomplished a great work.

It takes courage to examine ourselves with these questions:

How are my feelings and behavior determined by past injuries? Do I want to move beyond the pain and anger? How might I pray for the grace to take the next step in the forgiveness process?

Do I judge myself or others in any way? Can I see myself or others as God does?

Can I imagine a way to be free and to end the cycle of retaliation? What do I need to do to move in that direction?

Practice Nonviolence[9]

Taking the extraordinary path of forgiveness to even greater lengths, we come to the possibility of mercy and nonviolence. With forgiveness, we give up our anger or resentment against another, relinquishing our desire to punish or penalize the offender, and this sets us free. Forgiveness is the first step toward nonviolence. Mercy, as defined by Webster's *Dictionary*, is not only "a refraining from harming or punishing offenders, enemies, persons in one's power, etc.," but it is also "*kindness in excess* of what may be expected or demanded by fairness."[10] [authors' italics] Nonviolence includes forgiveness and mercy and more: it is an expression of love in action, refusing to participate in violence in any form, and changing evil to good.

Nonviolence means taking hold of the power of love and truth in an active, courageous manner, even in the face of suffering. It means remembering that we are all children of God, all equal, all deserving of reverence and care. Nonviolence means the refusal to cooperate with injustice or to be controlled by it, not by retaliating, not by becoming passive victims. The person who practices nonviolence is able to love the perpetrator of injustice while abhorring and confronting the injustice itself.

Nonviolence is often associated with civil disobedience, which is one expression of nonviolence. Civil disobedience involves peaceful, public resistance to government or institutional policy as a matter of conscience. But, in fact, nonviolence is much broader and includes anything we do that avoids harm to others and extends love. There are degrees of violence and degrees of nonviolence. Any behavior that fails to reverence any part of creation is violence, from the "microviolence of inattention" to the "macroviolence of the arms race and its satellite violences."[11] Any behavior that cherishes and protects all facets of creation is nonviolence, from the "micro-" nonviolence of simple harmlessness and appreciation to the "macro-" nonviolence of civil disobedience.

Nonviolent leaders such as Jesus, Gandhi, Martin Luther King, Jr., and Steven Biko modeled the willingness to disarm *first*, knowing that the "enemy" is not an enemy at all, but a brother or sister. This willingness to go beyond the "reasonable," "fair," instinctual reaction to an injury, and *to extend love*, seems dangerous and crazy. It can only happen when we have absolute faith that to love is to bring God into the situation, and if God is God, then love and truth will ultimately be victorious. The only alternative is dangerous and crazy: as Martin Luther King, Jr. has said, "The choice today is no longer between violence and nonviolence. It is either nonviolence or nonexistence."[12]

The core disciplines gradually lead us to forgiveness, mercy, and nonviolence. Violence is self-centered, rooted in fear, selfishness, and greed; nonviolence is an expression of God-centered love. Violence is willful, exclusive, and clings to control and possessions; nonviolence is an expansive, inclusive willingness to share. Violence means dualistically dividing people into categories of "we" and "they," projecting unloved, unwanted parts of ourselves onto imaginary enemies. Nonviolence means remembering that we all share the same spirit and that when we hurt someone else, we hurt ourselves.

Believing that love and truth will triumph in the end, regardless of short-term costs; being willing to disarm, to reconcile, to help, to heal, to create community; resisting injustice peacefully; practicing harmlessness toward all of God's creatures, even our "enemies"—this is the toughest kind of love.

Jesus exemplified the epitome of nonviolence during his arrest, trial, and execution. His simple statements of truth, his silences, and his integrity throughout his trial modeled nonviolent confrontation. Even in his extreme suffering and anguish, he practiced forgiveness and love and faithfulness, giving himself to God with his last words. But he was not defeated. Our hope lies in the knowledge that even death could not stop his love and truth and power and presence, nor has it stopped others who have lived out the same heroic nonviolence.

We are not all called to civil disobedience, but we are all called to nonviolence. We can practice harmlessness and mercy in smaller ways, daily and consistently. We can pay attention to how we are interacting with others, what we are doing, what we are using, how it affects other lives. Our actions can be characterized by generosity, rather than exploitation and selfishness; by love, rather than fear. We need to heal, rather than hurt, one another; to be in solidarity with those who are vulnerable, with those who are disabled, elderly, young, sick, poor, or exploited. We need to extend forgiveness and mercy in the face of injury in order to break the cycle of retaliation. We need to show reverence for all of creation, and we must remember that we are all brothers and sisters and that we are all equal. Consider the alternative.

We might ask ourselves:

Do I show disregard for creation or do I take care to cherish and protect it?

How do I choose to perceive persons with whom I have a conflict? Are my responses to them guided by mercy or by a desire for retaliation? How might I introduce compassion into a difficult situation where kindness has been lacking?

How do I identify with others who suffer injustice, disability, disadvantage, or who are vulnerable and dependent?

How do I treat myself? Am I my own worst enemy, or am I gentle with myself?

Take Care of Yourself

When we hurt others, we hurt ourselves. Conversely, when we care for ourselves, we care for others. In order to be truly helpful to others, we must attend to our own needs. This is the way of trust: I believe that my needs and gifts are interdependent with others' needs and gifts; that in giving what I have to offer, others will receive according to their need; and I trust that others will meet my needs with what they have to give. The birds of the air and the lilies of the field are cared for by God's magnanimous provision, and so are we, through one another.

Attending to one's own needs does not mean passively expecting others to know what we need and to provide it. It does mean making our needs known, asking for what we need, and being able to accept that the other may not be able to meet our need. We may have to try someone or something else. Attending to our own needs also means being able to respond to others' needs with a willing yes, or a self-honoring no, without feeling guilty.

Self-discipline and self-care are active expressions of self-love. Truly caring for one's self is self-love, and we find pleasure in it. Whether diet and exercise, a discipline of prayer, protecting personal boundaries, or any other form of self-care, the practice does not have to be an exercise of will, a militant "have to." We may discover more lasting pleasure in enjoying a cup of tea than in gorging ourselves with cookies, which can lead to self-loathing; more satisfaction in exercise than in chronic inertia. At other times, eating a cookie or lazing in a hammock may be an enjoyable, self-caring thing to do. It is a question of balance. We all need work, play, solitude, togetherness, physical activity, rest, prayer, food, touch, and the giving and receiving of love.

It is important to look to one's self for guidance, rather than to what others may think. We do this by taking responsibility for ourselves, using our own power, rather than giving it away and thus seeing ourselves as helpless victims of external circumstances. Nor can we allow ourselves to be guided by others' moods, expectations, or positive or negative feedback. The wisdom we seek is within ourselves.

Paying attention to feelings, relationships, and the need to be faithful to God within also results in loving interaction with others. In order to feel safe and secure in a relationship, those around us need to know that we have boundaries and also that we can be trusted to speak and act with integrity. If we consistently live out what we think, feel, and believe, we hope to encounter other people who are doing the same thing. This kind of interaction leads everyone concerned into greater awareness, as we correct our beliefs and behaviors in response to one another. This process requires us to extend ourselves, which results in growth.

Health promotion requires that we attend to every part of our lives: physically, through good nutrition, exercise, safety measures, stress management, and disease prevention; emotionally, by attending to feelings, neither resisting them nor holding on to them; spiritually, by creating space in our lives in which to listen to God, to pray, to discover our embodied beliefs, to find meaning, to reverence the Holy within us and around us; socially, by practicing integrity in relationships, and by maintaining good communication and mutual support. Health and wholeness also require service to others, caring for the environment, and some form of investment in the future—caring for children, creating art, planting a tree, working for peace and justice. The authors believe that all of these are human needs, and that by taking care of these needs, we take care of our world and enhance our own and others' growth.

Questions we might reflect on include:

Am I leading a well-balanced life? If not, what is missing? What do I want and need?

Do I feel powerful, powerless, or both? Am I afraid to let go of control? Am I angry that life seems out of control? Do I feel safe, open, and trusting of life, people, God?

Do I deny, suppress, or hang onto my feelings, or do I allow them? Do I let others know how I feel? Am I open to their response? Do I have clear boundaries in my relationships? Do I ask for what I need from others or do I expect them to know intuitively? Can I accept that others may or may not be able to meet my needs? Do I feel guilty when I do not want to meet someone else's needs?

How am I taking care of my physical well-being? My emotional well-being and my relationships? My spiritual life?

Make Commitments

Our individual wholeness depends on healing interaction with each other, giving and receiving, allowing ourselves to be changed. Commitment makes growth possible.

Give yourself to whatever seems life-giving now—to a friend, a family, a church, a cause, a project. The opportunities for commitment are endless. It may be a short-term commitment, such as a summer garden or an exercise program, or a long-term commitment, perhaps to a community of faith or caring for an elderly parent, or a lifelong commitment, such as marriage and family.

Making a commitment opens the way for life and relationships to change us. When the going gets rough—and it will—therein lies the opportunity for real learning and growth. Our commitment sees us through, enabling us to mine the healing potential of our situation, regardless of the final outcome. Without commitment, the temptation is to leave a difficult situation unconsciously or prematurely. (We are talking here about *challenging* situations in life, not violent, abusive, or dangerous ones that must be abandoned immediately.)

For example, we frequently hear comments such as these from persons involved in healing ministry: "I joined the healing group at my church, and I have just about had it with these people. There is so much competition for recognition of gifts, backbiting, and pettiness, I just don't get it. I thought we were supposed to be a healing community." Perhaps it is an example of divine humor, that when we commit ourselves to healing (or peacemaking, or making a positive contribution of any kind), we find ourselves in a situation in which healing, or peacemaking, or justice is desperately needed. It is so much easier to heal the world than it is to heal ourselves and our immediate network of relationships. The groups to which we commit ourselves are the teachers we need to get in touch with the unhealed, the violent, and the unjust within ourselves. This is how the world will become more whole, peaceful, and just.

We say more about the healing potential of committed relationships, in families and familylike groups, in chapter 9.

We might ask:

Am I willing to extend myself for the well-being of other people? Am I willing to open myself to be changed through interaction with others?

When do I feel a strong, clear sense of belonging?

When do I feel alienated? What can I do to move beyond the experience of alienation?

Live Simply

It is truly a gift to be simple, as the words of a familiar Shaker hymn tell us, for simplicity is the key to freedom and joy. We have come full circle in our discussion of core disciplines: simplicity is the *fruit* of all the disciplines we have discussed. And, paradoxically, it is the *foundation* of all the other disciplines, because it is rooted in the first— keeping God at the center. It enables us to embrace the other disciplines in a continuing spiral of personal growth, which results in increasing freedom and profound joy.

We usually think of economics and relationship to material possessions when we hear the term *simplicity*. We must "live simply so others may simply live." Our comfort cannot be built on the oppression of other people. The complexity of the modern world disguises the problem of exploitation. It distances us from the persons who are hurt by our personal and collective materialism. We Americans use far more than our share of the world's food supply and natural resources. We need to wake up and look at what we are doing, to question the justice of it, and to seek solutions. The complexity of our world also masks the solutions, so that our individual efforts seem futile. The personal decision to boycott products obtained through oppression, to share food with hungry people, to shelter homeless persons, to recycle materials, or to buy less may seem small in the face of enormous problems, but it is not ineffective. These choices are all outward manifestations of an inward reality, and this inward reality will change the world.

Simplicity involves more than economic life-style and relationship to material goods; it is the opposite of idolatry. Simplicity means keeping God as the center of our lives. In *Celebration of Discipline*, Richard Foster writes that the reign of God must be central in the spiritual discipline of simplicity:

> The desire to get out of the rat race cannot be central, the redistribution of the world's wealth cannot be central, the concern for ecology cannot be central. . . . Worthy as all other concerns may be, the moment *they* become the focus of our efforts they become idolatry.[13]

He goes on to say that when God's reign is genuinely central, this central commitment necessarily leads to concern for the environment, the poor, the equitable distribution of wealth, and the end of oppression. All of these concerns flow out of and constellate around one's central commitment to God's will.

For the individual, simplicity is the ultimate stress management technique—in simplicity there is no more need to defend one's accumulated wealth, or to prove one's self by accumulating more; no more need to block out satisfaction and happiness by wanting things to be different; no more work and worry spent on holding onto what we have, whether material goods, power, or people; no more insecurity; no more depending on "success" or "failure" for self-image; no more feeling powerless over what one does and why; no more nagging guilt about the consequences of one's choices. The person who puts God at the center enjoys life with hard-won, childlike wonder and spontaneous concern for others. The human spirit, set free from idolatry, compulsion, addiction, or attachment is able to soar.

The poet Robert Bly says, "the soul wants most of all to praise, and that the more things we can praise, the stronger we are."[14] We are happiest when God is first in our lives and everything else arranges itself around that reality, for then we are truly free to love, to praise, to be at one with others, to give from our strength, to receive in our need.

Jesus taught, "For where your treasure is, there will your heart also be."[15] Where is your heart? What concerns or possessions in your life interfere with your ability to love yourself, others, and God?

These ten disciplines lead us into contact with the river of life, swimming and floating *with* the current that carries us along. As we learn to live this way, we find that we grow, little by little, in gentleness, love, surrender, willingness, and true humililty. We can feel ourselves gradually relax into life. This way of being in relationship with life promotes awareness, empowerment, harmony, and freedom—all important ingredients of a whole and healthy life. This is healing: a process, rather than a destination; a movement toward wholeness, as we saw on the horizontal axis of the bent-axis model of well-being (chapter 1).

As we move into part 2 on caring for your body, we focus on specific expressions of self-care in the form of nutrition, exercise, and disease prevention. The wisdom of the body draws us to seek what is healthy for us. Our bodies and minds then reward us with pleasure in good food, good friends, a good laugh or a good cry, movement, and safety. Self-care increases the abundance in life and enables us to love others as we love ourselves.

Part 2

Taking Care
of the Body

Introduction

HEALTH AND CHANGE

A physician sees two people who want to quit smoking. The first, a 47-year-old woman, says "I know smoking is bad for my health and my boss is putting pressure on me to stop. I know I should quit, but I tried it once before and almost went crazy. I just don't think I've got the willpower to do it."

The second smoker is a 38-year-old woman who tells her doctor: "It's really an awful habit and I know my health will suffer for it. I don't like depending on it to relax. I know that it's time for me to stop, and I feel that with some help I can do it."

The second woman is much more likely to be successful at quitting. Why?

When we want to change a habit, we try to muster "willpower." Often the pressure to change our behavior comes from someone besides ourselves: a mother, husband, or boss who thinks we should be different.

Motivation, on the other hand, is based on incentives that originate *within* our selves. We don't need justification from others to do what we feel is right. Although we may need help to accomplish what we want to do, we do have control over our own actions and behavior. This doesn't make behavior change easy, but it does increase our chance of success.

It is not enough to be aware that we need to change. We must also be aware of the underlying reasons why we act as we do, what obstacles stand in our way, and what resources are available for help.

Health educators have developed models to explain health behavior. One of these, called PRECEDE,[1] states that there are *predisposing*, *enabling*, and *reinforcing* factors that influence behavior. *Predisposing* factors include knowledge, beliefs, values, and attitudes. Statements

115

such as, "This treatment won't do me any good," or "I have complete faith in my doctor," or "This illness is a punishment from God and nothing will help" are all examples of beliefs or attitudes that affect our health. *Enabling* factors include availability and accessibility of resources, such as the cost of a certain service, its location, and hours of operation. *Enabling* factors also encompass personal self-care skills, the ability to cook, for example. *Reinforcing* factors include the feedback from others regarding one's behavior change. For instance, a teenager might get positive feedback from his peers for starting to smoke. A woman who has lost weight may get negative feedback from family members or co-workers.

These factors influence whether we will initiate a behavior change and stick with it. It may be true that if someone wants to change badly enough he or she will find a way to do it. But most of us need support in initiating and maintaining new behaviors. If too many obstacles block our way, we are more likely to give up and fall back to familiar habits. Initiating a behavior change is not so difficult. We all know people who have quit smoking for a few days, dieted for a week or two, or started exercise programs that faltered after a month. The tough part of behavior change comes when we must *maintain* the new habit. Here we need skills to help us cope with temptation, frustration, stress, and depression.[2] Given these skills we can view lapses as opportunities for learning and use them in preventing a more serious relapse into the old behavior.

What causes us to *want* to change? Reasons for changing may be related to our perception of how a certain behavior contributes to personal risk of disease or death. No one is yet able to measure perception of risk and determine at what point we see a risk as a personal threat. In one family, all the adults quit smoking when the patriarch was diagnosed as having lung cancer. But in other families this does not happen. What is the difference? Ken Bakken once said that a person's decision to change depends on the degree of "uncomfortableness" he or she experiences. When we experience too much discomfort, we want to make a change. People are often motivated to change for the better. In this section we make practical suggestions on how to do that.

THE RISE OF CHRONIC DISEASES

The three most common causes of death in the United States at the beginning of the twentieth century were influenza and pneumonia, tuberculosis, and gastroenteritis, all infectious diseases. Today the leading causes of death are heart disease, cancer, and stroke, all chronic non-infectious diseases. Although influenza and pneumonia are still important causes of mortality and AIDS is claiming an increasing number of lives, infectious diseases have less impact in this country than in much of the rest of the world.

Researchers have identified certain characteristics that increase an individual's risk for chronic disease. Some of these risk factors are not modifiable: age, sex, and family history, for instance. A 65-year-old man whose father and brother have each had a heart attack is at much greater risk for heart disease than a 25-year-old woman with no family history of heart disease. The man's risk factors cannot be changed.

However, some risk factors are modifiable. These vary according to the disease. Modifiable risk factors in heart disease include smoking, high blood pressure, and a high serum cholesterol level. If the 65-year-old man also smoked, and had high blood pressure and high cholesterol, he could lower his risk of heart disease by eliminating these modifiable risk factors.

The first step on the path toward wholeness is being aware of the options available to us. Our state of health is influenced by, among other things, our diet, exercise, habits, and health practices, all of which can be modified. There is much that is within our power to change. We can choose among options to suit our own unique path.

5

Nutrition And Diet

Love is a fine thing, but love with noodles is even tastier.

Yiddish proverb

RECOMMENDED DIET FOR HEALTHY AMERICANS

Eating is a complex behavior. It is influenced by family and ethnic traditions, as well as by moral associations, religious customs, and personal preferences. Convenience, cost, habit, social pressures, and advertising also play a part. Nutritional needs often take a backseat to these other influences. However, because of the variety of foods available in this country, most of us could change our diets to more healthful ones that are also satisfying to us. We must first become aware of what constitutes a nutritious diet. Then we can incorporate changes into our lives slowly so they become permanent.

Though we all differ physically and have different nutritional needs, scientists have developed general guidelines for healthy people to maintain and promote health. Some of these guidelines are listed in the Recommended Dietary Allowances or RDAs, which are suggested levels of protein, vitamins, and minerals that meet the nutritional needs of healthy persons. Although we see the RDAs listed on many food labels, these recommendations were designed for populations and were not meant to be followed by individuals. Also, these guidelines do not advise people on what types of foods to eat less of or to avoid completely.

However, a few years ago, the US Department of Agriculture and the American Dietetic Association developed and published the "Dietary Guidelines for Americans," a list of seven recommendations based on scientific research.[1] These guidelines, which are designed to provide a nutritious diet and to protect against a number of diseases, are as follows:

1. Eat a variety of foods.
2. Maintain desirable weight.
3. Avoid too much fat, saturated fat, and cholesterol.
4. Eat foods with adequate starch and fiber.
5. Avoid too much sugar.
6. Avoid too much sodium.
7. If you drink alcoholic beverages, do so in moderation.

As a group, Americans consume an excess of calories, fat, salt, sugar, refined foods, and alcohol, and not enough complex carbohydrates and unprocessed foods. These dietary habits have contributed to epidemics of chronic disease in our country: coronary heart disease, cancer, high blood pressure, diabetes, cirrhosis, and stroke. By making the following specific changes in our diet we can decrease our risk of these diseases.

Eating a variety of foods usually ensures a balanced and adequate diet. It is not possible to get all the nutrients one needs from a single food or group of foods. We should thus eat fruits, vegetables, whole grain products, and beans and bean products. Many people also choose to eat dairy products and meats, although the nutrients in these foods can be obtained from other foods. Ovo-lacto-vegetarians avoid meat, poultry, and fish. They can generally meet all their nutritional needs through their diet, including iron from green leafy vegetables and whole grains and vitamin B_{12} from dairy products. Pregnant women, however, should consult a nutritionist to make sure that their diets are adequate. People who eat no animal products at all, including eggs and dairy products, are called vegans. They may have difficulty meeting their needs of vitamin B_{12} and calcium. Their diet may be supplemented with vitamin B_{12}-fortified soy milk or cereal, and they should eat nondairy foods containing calcium, such as green leafy vegetables, broccoli, and tofu. If a variety of foods is chosen, it is usually unnecessary to take vitamin supplements, except in special circumstances. If you have any questions regarding the adequacy of nutrients in your diet, you should consult a nutritionist.

Maintaining desirable weight is very difficult for many of us. The weight loss industry is huge and the manufacture of artificial sweeteners and "diet" foods is a booming business. Inappropriate weight gain is more complex than merely eating too much. We explore the problem of obesity later, but, in general, the dietary guidelines for avoiding obesity are included in these basic recommendations.

High levels of fat in the diet may lead to high serum cholesterol levels, and high serum cholesterol is a risk factor for heart disease. Lowering the serum cholesterol can reduce the risk of heart attack. Americans are advised to decrease the amount of fat, saturated fat, and cholesterol in their diets. For most people this means decreasing the amount of red meat, egg yolks, dairy products (especially cheese), and fried foods, and substituting fish, poultry, beans, and broiled, baked, or boiled foods. We discuss cholesterol and fat in more detail later.

Contrary to popular belief, eating starchy foods will not make you fat. Starches, or complex carbohydrates, have, ounce for ounce, less than half the calories of fats. The culprit is not the starch but the high fat sauces or spreads used with them. For example, the much maligned baked potato, besides being a good source of protein and fiber, has only about 100 calories. Add butter or sour cream and that can add another 200 calories, most of it from fat. Foods that contain complex carbohydrates, such as dried beans and peas, whole grain breads and cereals, and potatoes, are good sources of many essential nutrients and fiber. Dietary fiber (the part of plant foods that is not digestible by humans) is thought to be a useful class of food that helps prevent chronic constipation and may prevent colon cancer. Soluble fiber, found in oat bran, fruit, carrots, and beans, may lower serum cholesterol. Fruits and vegetables are good sources of fiber and starch. These foods contain simple carbohydrates, such as fructose, and other important nutrients, including vitamins. They should be eaten instead of "sweets," such as candy and sodas, that contain predominantly sugar and are devoid of nutrients. Fruits are also more nutritious than high-fat desserts.

Sugar is not an essential nutrient. It occurs naturally in some foods and is added to many processed foods in various forms (dextrose, high-fructose corn syrup, maltose, and sucrose are just a few). Sugar contributes to tooth decay and has little or no nutritive value, except for calories. Sugar should be used in moderation. The less we use it, the more we are able to taste the natural sweetness of foods, and have less need to sweeten them with sugar.

Sodium is an essential nutrient, but we generally eat much more than our bodies require. Sodium is found in table salt, preservatives such as sodium benzoate, and flavor enhancers such as monosodium glutamate (MSG). About a third of the sodium in our diets is provided by processed foods and another third is added by ourselves.[2] Our physical needs could be met by the sodium that is found naturally in foods, and we could do without table salt and all the salt in processed and preserved foods. For many people, reducing dietary sodium will lower their blood pressure. So it is best not to get used to high salt content in foods. The recommendations are to substitute spices for salt, cook with little or no salt, add little or no salt to food at the table, use low sodium products, and limit intake of salty foods. As with sugar, the less salt you eat the less you will find you want.

Alcoholic beverages are high in calories and low in nutrients. Drinking in moderation does not appear to cause any harm in most adults as long as it does not lead to alcoholism. The level of alcohol use that constitutes moderation is subject to debate but is generally considered to be one to two standard-size drinks daily. Heavy drinking is associated with malnutrition, cirrhosis of the liver, certain types of cancer, and motor vehicle injuries, as well as psychosocial problems. Pregnant women are advised to refrain from drinking altogether, since alcohol has been shown to cause birth defects.[3] Alcohol may also be a factor in high blood pressure and obesity and may be used as a substitute for foods that have more nutrients.

In addition to these recommendations, St. Luke Health Center has developed suggestions on nutrition and diet for healthy Americans. We advise that people eat fewer animal products, especially meat. Vegetarians tend to have lower blood pressure and lower serum cholesterol levels as well as lower rates of obesity and diabetes, all of which are risk factors for heart disease.[4] Although the evidence is not conclusive, vegetarians may also have a lower risk of lung and breast cancer and of osteoporosis, kidney stones, and gallstones.[5]

We also recommend that products containing caffeine be eliminated from the diet (e.g., coffee, black tea, many sodas, and chocolate). Caffeine stimulates the cardiovascular and nervous systems and can be addictive. Its side effects may include palpitations, sleeplessness, and nervousness. Caffeine can raise blood pressure and cause disturbances of heart rhythm. It can also aggravate peptic ulcers. Withdrawal from caffeine may cause headaches, drowsiness, depression, and lethargy, but decreasing the amount of caffeine gradually can minimize these symptoms.

We also suggest limiting foods with artificial additives, which are sometimes used to prevent bacterial contamination. Such additives may, however, be harmful. For instance, nitrites used in processed meats are transformed in our bodies into nitrosamines, which are carcinogens.[6] Other less dangerous additives are not always necessary. We miss the good flavor of natural foods when we eat them with so-called flavor enhancers, such as MSG. Fresh foods prepared with natural accents, such as herbs and lemon juice, are usually more flavorful.

Finally, we recommend that food be prepared and handled with respect, that it be eaten slowly and intentionally, and that a thankful attitude be maintained with respect to the people and processes that go into providing food. What and how we eat reflect how we feel about our bodies and their needs. But above all, we should maintain a realistic perspective. Moderation is the key. The point is to follow an optimal diet most of the time so that when we do eat something that is not "good" for us, it is a treat and not a reason to feel guilty. After all, eating should be enjoyable. Having a sense of humor about ourselves helps us to return to our good eating habits with a sense of renewal and satisfaction.

SPECIAL DIETS: LOW-SALT, LOW-FAT, FOOD SENSITIVITIES

Special diets are often advised because of certain medical conditions. We will discuss here some of the more common diets associated with the treatment of disease.

People who have high blood pressure (hypertension) and certain types of kidney and heart disease are usually advised to restrict their sodium intake. These conditions can be helped by dietary changes. As mentioned before, sodium is found in table salt (sodium chloride), the preservatives sodium benzoate and sodium nitrate, MSG, baking powder, and baking soda.

Studies have shown that populations that use a lot of salt, the northern Japanese, for instance, tend to have a higher proportion of hypertensives, whereas societies that use little salt have very little high blood pressure.[7] Studies of individuals in industrialized countries, however, have not shown that salt ingestion *directly* causes hypertension.[8] There is uncertainty as to whether deficiencies of certain other minerals, such as potassium, magnesium, and calcium, may also contribute to high blood pressure.

A low-salt diet is one of the nondrug therapies available for people with hypertension. Recommendations include eliminating salt in cooking, except where absolutely necessary, and not using the salt-shaker at the table. Lemon juice and various herbs and spices (although not soy sauce, onion salt, or garlic salt) are palatable substitutes. Foods high in salt should also be avoided. These include many processed foods and snack foods, such as pretzels and chips. Foods containing sodium nitrate, such as cured meats, and those with MSG, such as Chinese food, should also be limited or avoided altogether. We encourage you to read labels on packaged foods. Companies must follow certain rules in order to call their product "low sodium" or "no sodium." Although food manufacturers are not required to list the amount of sodium on their labels, many are now doing so to attract consumers who are concerned about their sodium intake. Lists of foods that people with hypertension should and should not eat are available from the American Heart Association, Blue Cross/Blue Shield, and the American Dietetic Association.

Heart disease is the number one killer in the United States. Diabetes is also among the top 10 causes of mortality. Obesity is a widespread problem among adults and adolescents and is becoming more prevalent in children. Diet is thought to contribute to a number of types of cancer. Dietary intervention in the form of a low-fat diet can be useful to prevent and/or treat all of these conditions.

Americans eat about 40 percent of their calories as fat. The American Heart Association currently recommends that fat constitute no more than 30 percent of total calories. Dietary fat normally consists of saturated, polyunsaturated, and monounsaturated fats. These words refer to the chemical structure of the fat, that is, how many hydrogen atoms are attached to the carbon chain.

Americans also consume nearly 500 milligrams of cholesterol per day; the current recommendation is no more than 300 milligrams. Since cholesterol is not soluble in blood, it must be transported in "packages" composed of fats (lipids) and proteins, called lipoproteins. Low-density lipoprotein (LDL) is associated with an increased risk of coronary heart disease, whereas high-density lipoprotein (HDL) may protect against heart disease.

It is recommended that *saturated* fat comprise no more than 10 percent of total calories, because saturated fat causes the greatest rise in total and LDL-cholesterol, greater than dietary cholesterol itself causes. Saturated fats are generally solid at room temperature. They include all animal fats, such as butter, lard, beef tallow, and chicken fat, as well as tropical oils. (See Table 5-1.) *Polyunsaturated* fats decrease LDL- and HDL-cholesterol, but LDL is decreased to a greater extent. The American Heart Association recommends that these fats comprise up to 10 percent of total calories. Polyunsaturated fats have more hydrogen atoms than saturated fats and are usually liquid at room temperature. They include most vegetable fats *except* coconut, palm, and hydrogenated vegetable oils. *Monounsaturated* fats, such as olive oil, also decrease LDL-cholesterol but without lowering HDL and should provide 10 to 15 percent of total calories. The current recommendations are to use polyunsaturated and monounsaturated oils whenever possible, to avoid saturated fats, and to lower the total intake of fat.

Cholesterol is found only in animal products: meat, poultry, fish, eggs, and dairy products. Cutting down on these foods helps lower blood cholesterol.

In many instances, foods with both high saturated fat and cholesterol levels are meats and dairy products. By decreasing the consumption of these two food groups or by substituting low-fat alternatives, such as broiled fish, legumes, and low-fat dairy products, the blood cholesterol can usually be brought down. A number of books are available today that explain how to lower cholesterol with diet.[9]

Case Study

Andrew was 27 years old when he started to develop pain and stiffness in his lower back. He attributed the symptoms to "old age" and ignored them. In the next couple of years, however, the pain worsened and he found it increasingly difficult to move his neck fully. Andrew saw a physician who diagnosed ankylosing spondylitis, a severe, progressive form of spinal arthritis. He was put on anti-inflammatory medications that helped the pain but did nothing to retard the progression of the disease.

When Andrew came to St. Luke Health Center five years after his diagnosis he had pain and stiffness in his upper and lower back and neck. There was limited motion of his spine in all directions and evidence of muscle spasm in the upper and lower back. As part of Andrew's evaluation he was asked to keep a food diary for a few days that revealed that he was eating large amounts of processed foods, dairy products, fried foods, meat, and foods with a lot of refined sugar. He was advised to cut down on, or better, to eliminate

TABLE 5-1.

Saturated, Polyunsaturated, and Monounsaturated Fats

High Saturated, Low Polyunsaturated

coconut
palm kernel
beef tallow
palm
lard
butter
hydrogenated oils

High Polyunsaturated, Low Saturated

safflower
sunflower
corn
soybean
cottonseed

High Monounsaturated, Low Saturated

canola
olive
peanut

Source: US Department of Agriculture; cited in Jane E. Brody, "Personal Health," *New York Times*, December 7, 1989.

these foods and was told what kinds of substitutions he could make for a healthful diet. He also began an exercise program, received massage therapy, and continued his medication. In the next few weeks, he found that by eliminating dairy products and foods with refined sugar from his diet his pain diminished. He found that the diet, massage, and exercise gave him a degree of control over his symptoms that he had never before experienced.

Medical experts disagree about the role of food in allergies and sensitivities, but at St. Luke Health Center we have found that foods commonly cause symptoms in susceptible people. These symptoms can include rashes, such as eczema and hives, diarrhea, asthma, exacerbation of joint pain in arthritis, and sinus congestion.

When a person came to the Health Center with one or more of these symptoms, one of our recommendations for the person was to keep a food diary, including physical symptoms, for a number of days. The physician or nutritionist then examined the diary and made suggestions about the elimination or substitution of certain foods. In many cases the symptoms abated or were eliminated when the offending foods were removed from the diet.

Common offenders are dairy products, citrus fruits, shellfish, eggs, and foods with a high refined sugar content. A number of scientific studies have been done that support the link between food sensitivities and various physical symptoms.[10]

Certain foods may also affect a person's emotional state. We have found that people who eliminate specific foods, especially those foods with high sugar content and few nutrients ("junk food"), such as sodas and candy, sometimes report that they feel more energetic. Eliminating these foods will cause no harm, since they provide few if any nutrients. However, if you think that other foods may be contributing to your emotional or physical symptoms, be sure to consult a qualified nutritionist before eliminating a food to ensure that your diet remains wholesome.

Any significant dietary modification requires the cooperation of the person who buys and prepares the food and those who share mealtimes. Dietary intervention is best initiated with the participation and understanding of all the individuals involved. If you see a nutritionist or physician for dietary counseling, try to include these other people in the sessions so they can become familiar with your diet and help you follow it.

OBESITY

Throughout history people have made moral judgments of others with diseases. "Leper" describes someone with leprosy but also means an outcast or pariah. In the nineteenth century people who suffered from consumption were thought to have "romantic" personalities. Today sufferers of AIDS are viewed by some as "licentious." Probably the most widespread disapproval of an illness in our society, however, is that associated with obesity. Obesity, like leprosy, tuberculosis, and AIDS, may be viewed simply as a condition in need of treatment for purely medical reasons in order to relieve the suffering of the afflicted individual or to prevent future complications. However, this is rarely the case. Most people feel either disgust at an obese person's apparent lack of self-control, or pity for his or her apparent lack of self-esteem. The truth is that all human beings are wounded. Obese persons cannot hide their incompleteness as easily as others can.

Most people in our society find obesity to be aesthetically unpleasant. Those who want to lose weight are usually trying to fit into an ideal of beauty, and not because obesity is dangerous to their health. So we cannot address the problem of obesity from an entirely medical perspective but must take into account the psychosocial aspects as well.

However, we first define obesity medically and discuss its health implications. The National Institutes of Health Consensus Development Conference on the Health Implications of Obesity defined obesity as "an excess of body fat frequently resulting in a significant impairment of health."[11] It also stated that "an increase in body weight of 20 percent or more above desirable body weight constitutes an established health hazard. Significant health risks at lower levels of obesity can present hazards, especially in the presence of diabetes, hypertension, heart disease, or their associated risk factors."[12] Various tables have been developed that give ranges of desirable body weights according to height, age, sex, and frame size. One of the more popular tables was formulated by the Metropolitan Life Insurance Company. These tables will give you an idea if you are "overweight" but do not tell you if you have excess body fat. Some athletes have increased muscle mass and so appear to be over their desirable weight according to the tables. To find out if you have too much body fat, pinch the skin on the abdomen, under the upper arm, or below the shoulder blade. If you pinch more than one inch of skin then you probably have too much fat. This measurement can be done more accurately by a physician or exercise physiologist who uses skin fold calipers.

Obesity has a variety of adverse effects on health. Perhaps the most widespread effect is the psychological suffering it causes. The self-esteem of many people (especially women) has been affected because their bodies do not conform to the ideal of beauty in our society. Anorexia nervosa and bulimia are well-known eating disorders, and dieting is a constant preoccupation (or occupation) with a large proportion of the population. Our judgments of a person's beauty, sexual appeal, and competence are influenced by that individual's body size. Since there are approximately 35 to 40 million obese individuals in the United States, these problems are widespread.

In addition to the psychological effects of obesity, definite physical consequences often occur. High blood pressure and high serum cholesterol are two to five times more common in obese individuals compared to nonoverweight persons. These conditions are risk factors for heart disease, and both can be reduced by weight loss. Diabetes is about three times more common in overweight than in nonoverweight individuals, and weight reduction may reverse the problem of glucose intolerance in the diabetic.[13]

The relationship of obesity to coronary heart disease is less clear, but the latest research shows that the distribution of fat deposits may be a better predictor of heart disease than the degree of obesity, because excess fat in the abdominal area is more often related to heart disease than are fat deposits in the thighs or buttocks.[14]

Certain cancers have been associated with obesity, including cancer of the colon, rectum, and prostate in men, and cancer of the gallbladder, breast, uterus, and ovaries in women.[15]

Excess body weight results when the number of calories consumed surpasses the number of calories expended over a prolonged period of time. Simply stated, we eat more than we burn up day after day. Inherent biochemical causes of obesity, such as reduced thyroid activity (hypothyroidism) or excess cortisol excretion (Cushing's disease) are rare. More often obesity is caused by eating too many calories and/or not exercising enough. When an overweight person sees a doctor about losing weight, usually a diet of a certain caloric count is prescribed and the individual is advised to increase his or her activity. This approach rarely works over the long term, however.

The problem with diets, both doctor-prescribed and popular-press, is that they are viewed as temporary periods of deprivation in order to achieve the goal of weight reduction. When the goal is reached the individual is allowed to eat "normally" again. At this point most or all of the weight is usually gained back. This roller-coaster effect creates a situation that may be more dangerous to one's health than being obese and staying that way.

Obesity tends to run in families. Recently published evidence shows that heredity has a substantial influence on an individual's tendency toward obesity.[16] Some people seem to have a genetic predisposition to gain weight as fat rather than as muscle. However, in spite of this evidence, weight reduction is not a hopeless cause. A decrease in calories coupled with an aerobic exercise program of progressive difficulty often results in sustained weight loss if the exercise is continued.

Caloric restriction is never as easy as simply eating less. Food has many meanings in our lives. Obesity usually serves a legitimate need in a person's life that must be met a different way in order for a diet to succeed; habitual behaviors need to change; and there may be addictive elements to overeating.

Food carries many symbolic meanings for all of us. It is sometimes seen as a way to receive comfort, to assuage guilt, and to reward ourselves. When we give food to others we may see it as concrete evidence of our love or use it to manipulate people. Food has become more than just the fuel needed to sustain our bodies for necessary work.

Obesity can be used to avoid relationships or uncomfortable situations, or to remain dependent. If I am fat, I am therefore ugly and I won't have to deal with dating and sex. Or, I am really a nice person, but no one likes me because I'm fat. Or, the only way I can get anyone to pay attention to me is through my disability, which is lack of self-control and obesity. Often the individual is not aware of the feelings underlying the weight problem. However, if permanent weight loss is to occur these feelings need to be brought to the surface and explored.

Various types of interventions can be used to treat obesity in addition to diets. People who have difficulty losing weight on their own are often successful when they have the support of a group, such as Weight Watchers, TOPS, or those supervised by a physician or nutritionist. Together they discuss common difficulties and receive emotional assistance when needed. Sometimes exercise is a part of the regimen.

Recently, behavior modification has become a popular way of changing eating habits. This technique requires that an individual become aware of current eating behaviors, such as frequent eating while watching TV or snacking right out of the refrigerator, by keeping a diary of eating habits. The person then introduces different behaviors. These might include shopping only with a list, never buying items not on the list, eating only when seated at a table with a plate and utensils, putting the fork down between each bite, and always leaving food on the plate. This method takes the emphasis off the caloric content of foods and alters a person's eating behavior permanently so that fewer calories are eaten and the person loses weight.

Sometimes psychotherapy is useful to identify underlying reasons for overeating and weight problems. And though it can also help improve a person's self-esteem and change his or her role as "victim," psychotherapy alone is probably not enough to lead to permanent weight loss.

Another approach sees overeating as an addictive disorder, not unlike drug abuse or smoking. This method of intervention, used by

Overeaters Anonymous, views food as the addictive substance and helps individuals deal with overeating, rather than emphasizing initial weight loss. Unlike diets, support groups, and behavior modification, this approach views food as merely nutritional and seeks as its primary goal the elimination of compulsive eating behavior. Rehabilitation, brought about by changing life-style, using constructive coping techniques, and providing rewards other than food, is the key to this method.

This approach can present difficulties, however. Unlike drugs, alcohol, and cigarettes, food is necessary for life and cannot be abstained from completely. It is also socially acceptable to overeat, at least in certain situations, and very few people will be accused of gluttony if they do so.

At St. Luke Health Center, we have used a combination of these approaches for people who wished to lose weight or control their addiction to food. No one was given a diet. Rather, feelings and ideas about food were first elicited and then the individual kept a food diary for five to seven days, listing not only the food eaten but also physical activity, emotional states, and unusual stresses. The diary was then evaluated by a nutritionist or physician who made observations about types and amounts of foods eaten, degree of physical activity, triggers to eating or bingeing, and the uses of food for other than nutritional purposes. The practitioner then suggested appropriate ways to help the individual, perhaps periodic individual visits, group support, counseling, exercise, behavior modification, or rehabilitation, or a combination. The goal is to change a person's relationship to food permanently so that in the long run the risk factors for disease are reduced and the potential for a healthy life is improved.

NATURAL FOODS

By "natural food" we mean food that is in an unrefined state with all its original nutrients and no added preservatives and flavors. This does not preclude changing the form of the food, as when milk is made into yogurt or soybeans are made into tofu. Often these "natural" types of transformations increase the nutrients found in the foods. This is different, however, from combining sugar and water, adding ascorbic acid and a small amount of fruit juice, and calling it a nutritious fruit drink with lots of vitamin C.

Fifty years ago Americans ate a diet of fresh, unprocessed foods, with less meat, sugar, and fat.[17] More fresh vegetables, fruits, and complex carbohydrates were consumed. Now the American diet contains a much greater proportion of processed foods. These include canned foods, such as soups, vegetables, meats, and fruit; frozen foods, such as vegetables, dinners, and ice cream; and refined foods, such as white flour, potato chips and other snack foods, sugar, and packaged desserts. These foods can make meal preparation easier and quicker, but they are often less nutritious than their unprocessed counterparts.

The refining process tends to reduce the nutrients and fiber naturally present in food. This results in foods that are high in calories but low in nutrition. Fortification of foods has helped eliminate the problems of vitamin deficiencies that cause rickets, pellagra, goiter, and other nutritionally related diseases. Sometimes, however, the nutrients and fiber that are removed cannot be completely restored by fortification, as in the case of breads and cereals. In addition, processed foods generally deliver higher amounts of fats, salt, and sugar. Although food processing has contributed to the apparent abundance of food: "Were it not for food refining, it is doubtful that the average American could consume 130 pounds of sugar and nearly 120 pounds of fat a year."[18]

Other potential dangers in our food supply exist: the use of antibiotics in livestock, the application of pesticides to fruits and vegetables, the addition of preservatives and other additives to packaged foods, and the bacterial contamination of foods. Antibiotic use in cattle feed has been shown to produce drug-resistant bacterial strains that can cause illness and sometimes death in humans.[19] Pesticides used on fruits and vegetables are potentially harmful to people because of their cancer-causing effects on laboratory animals.[20] Washing produce before eating does not always eliminate the chemical. Additives, such as sodium nitrite in cured meat and some food coloring, may produce cancer-causing substances (nitrosamines) in the body.[21] The food industry claims that these chemicals are necessary in order to produce palatable, attractive, safe food. However, it is not the consumer who profits from fatter cattle at the market. Pesticides are often used indiscriminately when a more modest amount would serve the farmer's purposes better and be less harmful to the environment.[22]

We need to look critically at the production methods used in our food supply. Do we really need blemish-free cucumbers, uniformly orange oranges, and bright red meat? Could we tolerate less aesthetically pleasing food in order to have a safer food supply? This is a choice many people are able to make. Supermarkets and groceries are beginning to respond to consumer demand for uncontaminated food. It is often possible to grow some of our own food or to buy food grown without chemical fertilizers or pesticides. If we believe that our bodies deserve wholesome, unadulterated food then we can send the message to the food industry by purchasing safe and healthful foods.

FASTING

We have discussed the components of a healthful diet and how food can promote or hinder the achievement of health. At times, however, *abstaining* from food can be healthful.

Fasting is undertaken for physical, political, or spiritual purposes. Fasting for physical reasons may foster the healing of an illness, enable weight loss, or prevent illness from occurring. Political fasts, or hunger strikes, serve to bring attention to a cause. And fasting has been used for thousands of years as a discipline to increase spiritual awareness.

An absolute fast involves taking in no food or drink, including water. This can be done for no more than three days. Another type of fasting allows the consumption of water but nothing else. And a third type permits the drinking of fresh fruit and vegetable juices. This type of fast can go on for 40 days, or more in unusual cases. Fasts can be undertaken by individuals or groups, such as church congregations during a process of discernment, or on the Jewish Day of Atonement and other fast days. Muslims fast during the day throughout the month of Ramadan.

All major religions recognize fasting as a discipline to enhance spiritual awareness. Fasts were undertaken by Moses, the prophets Elijah and Daniel, King David, Queen Esther, Paul, and Jesus. Mohammed and Buddha also fasted for spiritual purposes. Fasting done for spiritual reasons is seen as an additional way to worship God, not as a means of self-congratulation for undergoing a physical ordeal. Fasting can reveal to us the degree to which we are controlled by things and pointless habits. Once we are aware of our dependence on the superfluous in our lives, we are empowered to seek a simpler and more balanced way of living. The awareness process happens over many fasts. For a fuller discussion of the spiritual discipline of fasting see Richard Foster's book, *Celebration of Discipline*.[23]

If you have never fasted before, we recommend that you ask an experienced person to help you. You should begin with a short fast of twenty-four hours, starting in the evening and forgoing breakfast and lunch the following day. You might take in no fluids, or drink water or fresh fruit juices, whichever you prefer. You may feel hungry during the day. However, it is perfectly fine to continue your normal activities, as long as you are not under excessive stress. If you are a regular coffee, tea, or cola drinker you may have a headache because of caffeine withdrawal.

A person's mental or spiritual attitude is important during a fast. Before undertaking a fast you should determine why you want to do it. During the fasting period, then, you can focus on the meaning of the fast, rather than on the deprivation you are experiencing. This is also a good time to examine your eating habits if your diet has not been healthful.

After going on short fasts weekly for a period of time you may want to attempt a 36-hour fast, or fasting from three meals, such as breakfast, lunch, and dinner on a single day. For a longer fast (three to seven days is common), we suggest you consult a qualified person or refer to a book on fasting.[24]

Do not undertake a fast if you have diabetes or an active malignancy; if you are pregnant or breast-feeding; or if you are extremely undernourished. If you are contemplating an extended fast to alleviate a physical condition or if you take any kind of medication, consult your doctor before starting the fast.

Claims of disease remission and improved health have been made by practitioners of fasting. Although we are not in a position to evaluate these claims, we are aware that fasting can result in a greater sense of physical, emotional, and spiritual well-being.

SUMMARY

A poll conducted by the *New York Times* in late 1987 showed that most Americans have not changed their diets despite health warnings by the medical community and the government.[25]

We often depend on habit, custom, and convenience when making choices about food. We do not think too much about what we feed ourselves, or we do not think it will make much difference if we do.

There are ways of increasing awareness of the importance of food to our physical, emotional, and spiritual health without becoming obsessed with every detail of our eating habits. One example is the Jewish dietary laws (kashrut). One purpose of kashrut is to exercise, and hopefully gain control over, one of the basic activities of our lives—preparing and eating food. In effect, we are engaged in determining boundaries for ourselves within which we regulate our lives. The value of this is twofold. First, such self-control is in itself a form of personal growth. It is a paradoxical truth that through the acquisition of discipline and structure within an otherwise random and arbitrary life, freedom, spontaneity, and personal growth become possible. Second, such personal boundary-setting constantly confronts us with the knowledge and responsibility that we are, and must always be, the masters of our own lives—our selves and our bodies.[26]

It is not necessary to keep kosher in order to obtain the benefits of dietary discipline. Just as we can change our attitudes about time (see chapter 3), we can change how we view food. Eating can be a spiritual discipline when it is approached with deliberateness and reverence. It takes time, awareness, and forethought to make such significant changes. When we are able to put food, eating, and diet into proper perspective in our lives, then what we eat becomes an expression of the way we nurture our bodies and spirits.[27]

6

Health Promotion

A door pivot will never be worm-eaten, and flowing water never becomes putrid.

Chinese proverb

EXERCISE

Most movement experiences in our day-to-day lives generally do not improve our physical well-being, unless we have physically strenuous jobs. In our society such jobs are rare. Even the demanding jobs of housework and child care do not promote physical fitness. To improve and maintain an optimum level of fitness, we need to exercise. A well-rounded exercise program includes activities that promote flexibility, endurance, strength, balance, and coordination.

Stretching for Flexibility

Stretching reduces muscle tension and promotes relaxation. It helps improve awareness of one's body and increases the range of motion of the extremities. It is absolutely necessary to stretch before and after strenuous activities to warm up the muscles and to prevent injuries. Best of all, stretching, if done correctly, feels good. Just about everyone can stretch and it can be done at any time of day. To learn to stretch safely, we recommend that you consult a qualified fitness instructor or a reputable book.[1]

Aerobic Exercise for Endurance

Aerobic exercises are endurance activities that require oxygen for prolonged periods and improve the body's ability to deliver oxygen to the tissues. Exercising in short bursts does not necessarily produce aerobic fitness, since during short-term activities, such as sprinting, the muscles do not require oxygen. These are called anaerobic exercises. Aerobic exercises include walking, running, cycling, swimming, and aerobic dancing.

Aerobic exercise can provide more energy, more restful sleep, weight loss, stronger bones, greater ability to deal with stress, alleviation of mild depression, and decreased risk of heart disease. If you want to begin an aerobic exercise program and have not exercised in a number of years, are over thirty-five-years old, or have a chronic medical condition, consult a physician for an evaluation. This should consist of a health history, including family history of heart disease; dietary evaluation; a thorough physical examination, including assessment of the musculoskeletal system; and a serum cholesterol test. Your doctor may also recommend an exercise stress test, or other procedures appropriate to your age, sex, and physical condition.

Once you have received the go-ahead, you should choose an activity that you enjoy. It is difficult to do something that you don't like, week after week, and therefore easy for you to become discouraged and give up before you have experienced benefits. You may find it more pleasant if you exercise with someone else.

Start slowly. If it becomes too tiring too soon, the tendency will be to quit. To achieve aerobic benefit you will need to exercise three days a week, 20 to 30 minutes per session. We recommend starting at five to 10 minutes per session and increasing the duration gradually over a few weeks.

An aerobic exercise program consists of three phases: (1) warm-up, (2) aerobic exercise, and (3) cool-down. Warm-up activities include walking and stretching. Once the muscles are warmed up and flexible, they are less prone to injury and the aerobic phase can be started. The cool-down period should consist of at least five minutes of the same activities done in the warm-up.

To find out if you are achieving the optimum aerobic benefit from your exercise, calculate your target heart rate before you begin exercising and measure your heart rate during exercise and compare the two. To determine your target heart rate, you need to approximate your maximum heart rate by subtracting your age from 220. For a 40-year-old person, for example, the maximum heart rate is about 180 beats per minute. The target heart rate is 65 to 80 percent of the maximum. We usually recommend about 70 to 75 percent. With a maximum heart rate of 180, the target heart rate should be 126 to 135 beats per minute. At some point during and immediately after finishing aerobic exercise, check your heart rate by taking your pulse for 10 seconds and multiplying the result by six. If you have recently had a heart attack, have chronic heart or lung disease, or are taking medication you should check with your doctor first, since your target heart rate may differ from what would be calculated by this formula.

As your aerobic capacity improves you will need to exert yourself more to achieve the target heart rate. This means that your body is becoming conditioned and you are benefiting from your exercise.

Remember, if you want to start an aerobic program, consult your doctor, a fitness instructor, or an exercise physiologist, or read a book by a qualified author.[2] By starting out in an informed manner you will be increasing your chances of staying with the program and minimizing your risk of injury. You will also find, after about six weeks, that you will look forward to your exercise sessions as an enjoyable part of your routine.

Exercises for Strength

The most common muscle strengthening exercises are calisthenics and weight lifting. Calisthenics are activities such as sit-ups, push-ups, and pull-ups that do not involve any special equipment. Weight lifting is done using free weights, devices such as Universal Gym, or special machinery such as Nautilus. These exercises develop specific muscle groups through repetition and increased resistance. They increase muscle mass and tone but do not diminish fat deposits.

As with aerobic exercise, start out slowly. Weight lifting should be done under the supervision of a qualified instructor. If you have high blood pressure or heart disease you'll need the specific consent of your physician. These exercises can cause dangerous elevations in blood pressure or irregularity of heart rhythm.

Muscle strengthening exercises are best done as part of a program that includes aerobic exercise and flexibility training. These three types of exercise complement each other and allow a greater range of improvement with a decreased risk of injury.

Meditative Exercise for Balance and Coordination

Two meditative exercise disciplines that help develop and integrate our physical and spiritual lives are yoga and t'ai chi ch'uan. Yoga was developed thousands of years ago in India to enhance contemplation and prayer. It consists of body positions and methods of breathing that improve flexibility, balance, concentration, and strength. The cultivation of these physical and mental attributes helps develop spiritual energy. Yoga is said to contribute to rest, serenity, and peace of both body and soul, which creates receptivity to greater spiritual awareness.

T'ai chi, which was developed in ancient China, is a dancelike series of movements choreographed for health and self-defense. All forms of t'ai chi in existence today are based on the same principles. T'ai chi involves a designated series of movements, practiced in slow motion, which help develop balance, concentration, and stability. They help release tension and promote a state of relaxation. At a faster tempo t'ai chi can be used for self-defense and have aerobic benefits. The movements of t'ai chi originate in the center of the body. They are initiated by the mind rather than by muscular force. As in other martial arts, the movements are controlled by a tranquil spirit. Unlike other disciplines, t'ai chi creates a slow, continuous, and effortless meditation. Yielding is an important principle of t'ai chi. When attacked, the student is taught to yield, creating instability in the opponent, and making it easier to counterattack. This attitude of yielding can also be applied to an individual's mental and spiritual life, which leads to greater serenity and a sense of well-being.

Yoga and t'ai chi are best learned from experienced teachers rather than from books. It is important to seek out an instructor who teaches the technical skills and also imparts the spiritual attitudes of the discipline.

Case Study

Carl was 20 years old when he lost control of his motorcycle. The crash threw him 75 feet and knocked him unconscious. He was taken to a hospital where he was placed on a respirator. He was in a deep coma and his right side was paralyzed. After a month, his parents were told that he probably would not live. One month later he reacted to painful stimuli and opened his eyes.

After four years of physical, speech, and occupational therapy, and classes at a rehabilitation facility, Carl was able to get his driver's license and a job. He still had a severe limp, a contracture of the right arm, and slurred speech. He described himself as a workaholic who smoked, drank too much, and was overweight. At St. Luke Health Center, his massage therapist suggested that he try t'ai chi.

At first Carl noticed no progress with his disability, but after a year of study things began to change for him. He became "more aware" of his body and felt "more life" than even before the crash. His family commented on his improved balance and gait. He stopped smoking and drinking and lost weight.

More recently, Carl has noticed changes in the way he thinks and has become more disciplined in his spiritual life. He practices t'ai chi every day and is no longer officially considered disabled.

Carl's t'ai chi instructor has noticed that his balance and coordination have improved and his limp has diminished. Carl is also learning to yield in difficult interpersonal situations. In addition, he has greater self-esteem, which allows him to seek new challenges.

SMOKING

Smoking causes the greatest number of preventable deaths in the United States. Every year more than 350,000 people die from diseases related to cigarette smoking.

Smoking cigarettes can raise the risk of dying from a number of cardiovascular diseases, including heart attack, stroke, and clots in the aorta and other arteries. Lung cancer is the most common form of cancer in the United States, and 80 to 85 percent of the cases can be attributed directly to smoking. However, cancers in other areas of the body are also associated with smoking. These include cancer of the larynx (voice box), mouth, esophagus, bladder, pancreas, and possibly other sites.

Years of smoking can produce chronic obstructive lung disease (emphysema and chronic bronchitis). These illnesses make breathing progressively difficult, and can lead to continual use of oxygen and, eventually, premature death. Peptic ulcers are also more common in people who smoke.

These frightening statements about death and disease from smoking do not fully convey the suffering that individuals experience. Heart attacks can kill quickly or may cause long-term disability. Surgical treatment for various cancers may be disfiguring or debilitating. Chronic lung disease can literally cause a person to suffocate.

Why do more than 25 percent of all adult Americans continue to smoke? And why do 4,000 adolescents and children start smoking every day? No one likes the first cigarette. It is a habit that is learned. So the reasons for starting smoking involve more than taste and pleasure.

Most smokers start smoking by the age of 20. Adolescents who take up smoking are influenced by their friends and family members. They are especially likely to start if one of their older siblings already smokes.[3] Another contributing factor may be that about one-third of teenagers think there is no health risk associated with smoking.[4]

The addictive quality of nicotine makes quitting smoking difficult. Nicotine is a drug, which may be more addictive than heroin. It causes physical changes: increased heart rate, increased blood pressure, decreased appetite, and improved alertness. Abrupt withdrawal from nicotine will produce the opposite effects. Since smoking is also psychologically addictive, quitting may cause irritability, anxiety, depression, and sleep disturbances. Someone who has quit smoking may continue to crave cigarettes and some people report a desire for cigarettes years later when they are reminded of a pleasurable situation they associated with smoking. However, the craving for nicotine will diminish over time.

Still, tens of millions of Americans have quit smoking since the US Surgeon General first warned of the danger of smoking in 1964. More smokers are finding it inconvenient, if not stigmatizing, to smoke in public places. Nonsmokers' rights have been bolstered by the 1986 *Surgeon General's Report* that involuntary smoking causes disease, including lung cancer, in nonsmokers; that children whose parents smoke have more respiratory infections; and that separating smokers from nonsmokers within the same airspace does not eliminate exposure to smoke.[5]

Sadly, women are taking up smoking in increasing numbers and have been less likely to quit than men. If a woman smokes only one to four cigarettes a day, her risk of a heart attack is more than doubled. Smoking reduces a woman's fertility, increases the risk of miscarriage and of bleeding during pregnancy, and causes fetal growth retardation. Exposure to cigarette smoke during pregnancy may also affect a child's long-term physical, intellectual, and emotional development.[6]

So if you smoke, how can you help yourself enjoy a healthier life? About 95 percent of smokers who quit do it on their own without help from groups, physicians, or medications. However, about 90 percent of current smokers would like to quit but find it too difficult.

It therefore seems that those who still smoke have the most serious addiction and might benefit from outside intervention.

A number of different types of interventions are available. Voluntary organizations, such as the American Lung Association (ALA) and the American Heart Association (AHA), as well as commercial concerns offer smoking-cessation programs in group format. These classes usually meet once a week for a number of weeks and help participants discover their reasons for smoking, provide behavior modification techniques to help cut down or eliminate smoking, and teach ways to cope with temptations to resume smoking.

For those who do not wish to join a group, publications are available from the ALA, AHA, and the National Cancer Institute, which cover much of the material presented in classes. It is, however, up to the individual to choose which techniques would be most beneficial for him or her. This type of intervention takes more motivation since group support is not available.

A third alternative is nicotine gum, which must be prescribed by a physician. The individual must quit smoking on the day the gum is started. He or she chews a piece of gum slowly every time the urge to smoke arises. The gum keeps the blood level of nicotine up so the individual does not experience physical withdrawal symptoms. Eventually, the quitter must wean from the gum since it too can be addictive. Nicotine gum is most successful when it is combined with a behavior modification program to help the individual become a nonsmoker.

Other smoking-cessation interventions include biofeedback, hypnosis, acupuncture, and aversive conditioning. In aversive conditioning, the individual "oversmokes" so he or she becomes ill or associates smoking with unpleasant effects.

It seems that one type of intervention does not offer any particular advantage over any other. All types have similar abstinence rates at the end of one year. It does appear that the more often a person tries to quit the better is the chance for success. Predictors of success in long-term cessation include support from friends and family and the greater use of self-reward and problem-solving techniques. Also, those individuals whose physicians urged them to quit smoking were more likely to follow through.[7]

One other predictor of outcome is self-perception, that is, whether or not individuals see themselves as responsible for making changes and capable of maintaining the result. This attitude is true of any behavior change. Do we view ourselves as victims of outside forces or internal urges, or do we have control over what we do? Beating an addiction to tobacco is difficult to do, but it is not impossible.

Case Study

John came to St. Luke Health Center suffering from severe headaches, earaches, and a nervous stomach. He also reported feeling stressed. Fifty years old, married with five children, John worked two full-time jobs because he wanted to retire while he was still young.

John's visit with the physician revealed that his diet was poor and that he had smoked about one pack of cigarettes per day for the past 35 years. He had tried to stop smoking a couple of times, but he liked to smoke and couldn't stop. The physician prescribed nicotine gum for John and referred him for biofeedback training for the headaches and nervous stomach and to help him stop smoking.

The biofeedback therapist discovered that John had poor occlusion of his teeth and that he chewed gum almost constantly. The gum chewing aggravated the jaw problem and contributed to his frequent headaches, earaches, and upset stomach. The therapist discussed the bad effects of smoking with John. She told him that smoking was worse than sitting behind a bus and breathing in the exhaust fumes, and suggested that he visualize breathing in bus exhaust every time he took a drag on a cigarette.

John learned to do slow deep breathing and was told to practice it a number of times a day. He was also advised to cut down gradually on the number of cigarettes he smoked and was taught some behavior modification techniques.

A week later John decided to quit smoking. He chewed six to eight pieces of nicotine gum and practiced his relaxation exercises daily. He completely stopped chewing ordinary gum. Two weeks after he started biofeedback his headaches were gone. The relaxation training went on and John continued to practice at home. One month later he was chewing one piece of nicotine gum a day, and three months later he was off the gum completely. John was motivated to quit when he found out how smoking harmed his body and he was able to benefit immediately from the training in relaxation and behavior modification.

Smoking costs our society tens of billions of dollars each year in health care and decreased productivity, as well as personal loss to families. More young people could be deterred from acquiring the habit if we as a society decided that we needed to get serious about tobacco addiction and its severe consequences.

Smoking cessation is an individual effort, but as a society we can discourage smoking and encourage quitting in many ways. We can increase the excise tax on cigarettes, give discounts on life and health insurance to nonsmokers, ban advertising of tobacco products, and restrict smoking in public places.

ALCOHOL AND DRUG USE

Many Americans consider the issue of alcohol and drug dependency and its associated societal problems as one of the gravest issues we face as a nation. We explore the estimated magnitude of the problem; its effects on the individual, the family, and society; and strategies for its treatment and prevention.

Alcohol and drug abuse is defined as recurring physical, emotional, or social problems associated with alcohol or drug use, including the use of over-the-counter medications, prescription drugs, or illegal drugs. Symptoms of alcohol and drug dependency include tolerance, or the need for increased amounts of the drug to produce the same effect, and withdrawal symptoms when the intake of the drug is reduced or cut off.

Alcohol and drug dependency are now seen as two aspects of the same problem because most people with a dependency use more than one drug. However, research and treatment have traditionally been separate, according to the substance abused.

It is estimated that 5 to 10 percent of American adults abuse alcohol or are heavy drinkers. About 75,000 deaths per year are attributed directly or indirectly to alcohol, including medical illnesses, motor vehicle crashes, and mishaps such as falls, fires, and suicides. The use of alcohol can lead to medical complications, including chronic liver disease and cirrhosis, nutritional deficiencies, pneumonia and tuberculosis, brain damage, high blood pressure, heart disease, mental illness, sexual dysfunction, depression, various types of cancer, and fetal malformation.

Legal problems associated with alcoholism include arrests for driving while intoxicated and for violent behavior associated with excessive drinking.

Many experts believe that alcoholism is caused by a combination of factors. Certain people seem biologically prone to developing alcoholism because of the way their bodies metabolize alcohol. This tendency is reinforced by a culture that encourages the use of alcohol to relax, socialize, and decrease stress. Drinking, even excessive drinking, is a socially acceptable activity. Individuals at greatest risk of abusing alcohol are those with first-degree alcoholic relatives, those who undergo periodic stressful changes (such as people in the military and the unemployed), and adolescents.

The alcoholic individual has two characteristic features: an inability to control drinking and denial that there is a significant problem. Treatment begins by breaking down the denial, which is best achieved by confronting the individual with the medical diagnosis of alcoholism in an empathetic manner, and offering the alcoholic hope for recovery. Alcoholism is a disease, but recovery from it requires the individual to take responsibility for accepting treatment.

Recovery is an ongoing process. Abstinence from alcohol use can be achieved as an outpatient or in the hospital. Continued abstinence depends on the individual's involvement in either Alcoholics Anonymous or group psychotherapy. Relapses during the first two to three years of treatment are common. However, if they maintain treatment for this length of time, about 70 percent of alcoholics will successfully recover from their alcoholism.[8]

Statistics about drug abuse are hard to come by, but it is estimated that about 2.5 million Americans have a serious drug problem. Drug dependency costs our society from $10 to $47 billion per year. Drugs of abuse include: (1) narcotics, such as heroin, codeine, and Demerol; (2) barbiturates, such as Seconal; (3) tranquilizers, such as Valium; (4) stimulants, such as cocaine and amphetamines; and (5) marijuana. Those who abuse drugs are usually dependent on more than one, and like alcoholics, drug abusers experience tolerance and withdrawal symptoms. Symptoms of withdrawal can appear many years after the user has quit using drugs if a situation recurs that was previously associated with the individual's drug use. Relapse into drug use will often depend on the availability of the drug during this period of distress.[9]

Intravenous drug use can cause serious infections, such as hepatitis and AIDS. Any drug taken in overdose may result in death. Another problem associated with drug abuse is violent crime, which is committed either to obtain money to buy drugs or between rival drug dealers. Some people who abuse drugs are able to maintain a job, but eventually the craving for the drug will dominate the person's life and cause disintegration in the family and poor performance at work. As with alcohol dependency, legal problems may also occur with drug dependency.

Treatment of drug dependency is similar to treatment for alcoholism. Short-term abstinence is achieved either as an outpatient or in a treatment facility. Long-term abstinence depends on an involvement in group therapy or Narcotics Anonymous and on the availability of drugs in the person's environment.

For every person who has a chemical (drug or alcohol) dependency it is estimated that three to five other people are affected. These friends and family members will often adapt to the individual's dependency rather than confront the behavior. This adaptation helps preserve stability in the relationship, but eventually it may lead to emotional problems in the user's friends or relatives. When these psychological problems arise in a friend or relative, the individual is said to have a co-chemical dependency, or codependency for short.[10]

Adaptation by the codependent individual to the abusive behavior of the dependent person either enables or accepts the behavior of the dependent person. Enabling may take the form of denying that the person has a problem, covering up for him or her when there is trouble, or protecting the person from the consequences of his or her behavior, such as on the job or with the law.

As a result of this denial, codependent individuals may develop various physical and emotional symptoms that are not outwardly related to the family member's substance abuse. Codependents often have inadequate trust in their own perceptions and have little sense of self-worth. Effective treatment for a codependent person is similar to treatment for the dependent person. It includes acceptance by the individual that he or she is codependent as well as participation in a group such as Al-Anon, Alateen, or Adult Children of Alcoholics (ACOA). Individual or group psychotherapy is often also helpful.[11]

In addition to family members, codependency can be present in members of the helping professions, co-workers, and society at large. As individuals we help maintain an atmosphere that is conducive to substance abuse whenever we fail to confront someone who we know is misusing alcohol or drugs, when we put a positive social value on drinking or drug use, and when we stigmatize people with dependencies or people who abstain from alcohol and drugs.[12]

As with smoking, prevention strategies for alcohol and drug dependency often involve only the individual. However, society can do a great deal to address the broader policy issues in this area. For alcohol abuse these interventions would include educational programs (especially for children and adolescents), warning labels on containers, increased price of alcohol through taxation, counteradvertising, establishment of legal responsibility of bartenders for damage caused by an intoxicated patron, elimination of "happy hours," and an increase in the legal drinking age to 21.[13] Societal intervention for drug abuse could include an increase in the availability of treatment programs, early identification of users, and an increased funding for youth programs that would reduce the likelihood of drug use.[14]

For those who do not abuse alcohol or drugs, it is difficult to see how others can let their lives revolve around something so destructive for the short-term goal of feeling good (or not feeling bad). But if we look further, we see that the problem of addiction is pervasive in our society.

As consumers, we can be addicted to owning things, to possessing that which is "new and improved." Advertising, especially on television, makes anything that is not up-to-the-minute sound undesirable. And since new things get old so quickly we must constantly buy more new things to feel good. Eventually, feeling good because of what we own, rather than because of our inherent self-worth, may become the center of our lives. We may begin to measure our love for others by what we buy them and to measure our own value by what we possess. Just as a drug addict may desire the high associated with the drug, we may come to believe that buying and owning certain things can relieve our boredom. Eventually we may begin to ignore the spiritual side of our lives, to the detriment of ourselves, our families, and the world.[15]

Therefore, we cannot judge the drug abuser and alcoholic as "other." As consumers, we too have succumbed to an addiction, albeit a socially acceptable one. Would it be possible that by rejecting consumerist values and instead offering our children a model based on the inherent worth of the individual, we could also affect the general problem of addiction in our society and change the ethic that allows it to exist?

STRESS MANAGEMENT

Case Study

Ellen and Diane work for a large insurance company doing data entry. Their boss has said that if they achieve more than 85 percent of expected job performance they will receive a cash bonus, which would be adjusted to each percent of increase. After one month Ellen is working at 110 percent of expected output with an enthusiastic attitude and many plans as to how she will spend her bonus. Diane, on the other hand, is working at 105 percent of expected job performance and feels tired and achy all the time. She likes the extra money, but she wishes that her boss had never started the incentive.

Why is the same incentive seen as a challenge by one person and a stress by another?

As we discussed in chapter 2, stress is the reaction our bodies exhibit when we are confronted with change. The situations that trigger that physical reaction are called stressors. Ellen and Diane experience the same stressor, but only Diane would say that she is "under stress."

Most of us associate stressors with death, divorce, debts, and excessive responsibilities. But positive experiences can also result in the stress response . A promotion, wedding, birth, and vacation are stressors that may elicit similar reactions in us. Stress, then, can be caused by any change in the expected routine.

Our experience of stress is determined by our personal emotional reaction to it. This gives us two ways to manage stress. The first is by changing the nature of the stressor itself, and the second is by changing how we perceive the stressor intellectually and emotionally.

Some situations, such as loss of a loved one, are impossible to change. But many other, more common stressors in our lives can be modified.

Case Study

Henry was a 62-year-old manager who had been employed at a large corporation for 15 years. He was involved in a motor vehicle crash and had injured his back. A year later, he was still experiencing debilitating back pain. At St. Luke Health Center, he received massage and physical therapy and his back pain improved considerably. However, he hit a plateau in his progress after about one month and continued to have some pain almost every day for which he took anti-inflammatory medication. When this happens in body work, the cause of the block is often emotional, not physical. In Henry's case, the massage practitioner learned that he was tired of his job and wanted to quit. Upon inquiry, Henry discovered he was eligible to retire. A financial adviser helped him plan for the future. Three months later Henry decided to retire and his back pain resolved.

Henry had much more control over his situation than he thought and he found a workable option. This is often the case. It is easy to complain about the stressors in our lives but difficult to look for solutions to the problems. Sometimes all that's needed is to talk to the people who elicit the stress response in us, be they our supervisor, spouse, child, or neighbor. Other day-to-day problems we face, such as too much or too little work to do, who will cook dinner, the family budget, or late night noise, might be alleviated this way. If we are assertive about our personal needs, the people we must deal with are often agreeable about changing the situation. And the change may benefit more than one person.

There are times when change may not be possible in a given circumstance. You feel that you are overworked and let your supervisor know this. The supervisor says that she is under pressure by her boss, and if you don't do the work you'll be out of a job. What do you do then? You may have a number of options. You could look for another job, spend more time at work, or speak to someone in senior management or your union (if your workplace is unionized) about your situation.

Employers have a legal and ethical responsibility to provide a healthful work environment for their employees. Stress can damage health, and although it is not as obvious a hazard as coal dust, stress is much more pervasive. If you find that what you are experiencing is common in your worksite the employer should help alleviate the problem. Some companies tell employees that stress is their problem and that they should learn time management and relaxation techniques to deal with the stress. Others are willing to work with employees to improve the situation. These companies often find that when they respond to their employees' needs, morale, productivity, and attendance improve.[16]

The keys to initiating changes in the external environment are an awareness of what is causing the stress, a willingness to work at a solution, and an idea of the options available to you.

Even under these circumstances companies, relatives, or others may be unwilling to make changes. What are your alternatives then? As we mentioned before, events are not inherently stressful. The stress we experience comes from the way we perceive and interpret the external world. Diane and Ellen, in our previous example, had completely different reactions to the same situation. The incentive itself is a neutral circumstance. But only Diane experienced stress because of it. Because our perceptions color our reactions, if we change our perceptions, our reactions may be less detrimental to our health and well-being. This does not produce a frivolous attitude about important things. When we utilize stress-management techniques we retain the capacity to care about a situation without experiencing the debilitating emotional and physical effects of stress. Very often this allows us to deal more effectively with the situation itself.

Another effective stress-management technique is talking to people we trust. When confronted with a difficult situation, it is often helpful to talk it out with a spouse, other relative, or friend. Expressing our feelings to a caring person will not change the stressor, but it may defuse the stress reaction so we can emotionally leave the situation and go on to something else.

In cases in which an understanding confidant is unavailable or the situation causes more than a normal amount of stress, it can be helpful for you to speak to a counselor or psychotherapist about the problem. Choose a person who knows how to listen actively, rather than someone who only wants to offer advice (friend or professional).

One constant source of stress for many of us is the lack of time. We feel as though we rush around from one activity to another, trying to fulfill our obligations to our family, our job, our friends, and (often last) ourselves. We don't think about what is essential in our lives and what could be postponed or eliminated. In this situation it can be helpful for us to keep track of our activities for a few days to find out how much we are really doing, list those activities according to their importance, and then organize our day more efficiently. We can often find alternatives by asking others to share responsibility, by cutting back on our own and others' expectations, or by simply eliminating the activity for a while to see what happens. By simplifying our life, we can spend more time in those endeavors we actively choose to pursue.

Case Study

Greg was a 38-year-old man, mildly mentally retarded, who had worked in a sheltered workshop for 15 years. The workshop was closing and Greg had to find a job elsewhere. He brooded constantly about the change and feared that he wouldn't be able to cope with it. The impending disruption became a crisis to him. When he came to St. Luke Health Center, he talked about nothing else. Anxiety had taken over his life. We reminded him that he had coped with other changes in his life and listed some of them for him. Then we suggested that he try to view this change as a challenge rather than a source of stress. We emphasized his ability to get along with people and make friends, his talent for learning manual skills, and the possibility of earning more money.

* * *

We were encouraging Greg to think differently about his situation in order to relieve his stress. This is a cognitive technique in stress management. It does not change the situation but does alter our perception of it. For instance, if our boss tells us we botched an assignment and we take the criticism as a personal attack, then we'll certainly feel stressed and angry. On the other hand, if we consider the feedback as constructive, we can use it in improving the way we handle the assignment.

This technique is useful when other people fail to live up to our expectations. They may be strangers, drivers who cut us off, or store clerks who ignore us, business associates who do not return our phone calls, or neighbors who don't cut their grass. These little annoyances can add up if we let them. It is harder for us to cope with serious stressors when we're depleted physically and emotionally by the minor ones. Is it worth the energy for us to get worked up about such nuisances? If we can consciously tell ourselves not to dwell on these issues, eventually the irritants will have little impact on us. Dr. Robert Eliot, a cardiologist who works to prevent heart attacks, says it succinctly: "(1) Don't sweat the small stuff, and (2) It's all small stuff."[17]

Humor is a great stress-management technique. It is impossible to be distressed and laugh at the same time. (We're talking about a real belly laugh, not a nervous laugh.) Humor helps us take ourselves and others less seriously and allows us to slip up and have fun doing it.

Another way of dealing with and preventing the stress reaction is through relaxation. This is not the same as recreation. Some forms of recreation help us feel relaxed, but they do not produce the "relaxation response," which is essential to benefiting from these techniques.

The relaxation response is elicited when a person engages in meditation, centering prayer, autogenic relaxation, or progressive relaxation. It causes specific physiologic changes: a decrease in respiratory rate, heart rate, muscle tension, and sometimes blood pressure. This is the direct opposite of the fight-or-flight response to stress. These changes occur during sleep but not as quickly as in the relaxation response. The response increases the intensity and frequency of alpha brain waves, which are associated with states of deep relaxation.

To elicit the relaxation response, one must repeat a word, sound, phrase, prayer, or muscular activity and one must passively disregard everyday thoughts when they occur and return to the repetition.[18] Most techniques suggest that you sit upright with your feet on the floor or sit in a semireclining position. It is also possible to achieve the relaxation response during exercise. Usually it is helpful to say the repetition silently to yourself with each exhalation, or you may simply concentrate on your breathing. It is necessary to have a passive attitude regarding external disturbances and distracting thoughts. Whenever these thoughts enter your mind, take note of them and let them go. Then return to the repetition of your word or phrase. Do the relaxation in a quiet place to minimize distractions. Once you become proficient at eliciting the relaxation response, it can be done almost anywhere. Systematic relaxation of muscle groups is another technique that can help quiet the mind and provide deep relaxation.

Biofeedback teaches a person how to elicit the relaxation response. Electrodes are placed on a certain muscle group, usually the forehead, and are attached to a machine that converts degree of muscle tension into an auditory or visual message. The higher the degree of tension the more frequently the light flashes or sound beeps As the student achieves the relaxation response, the muscles relax and the frequency of the beeping or flashing diminishes. The student is capable of voluntarily controlling the level of muscle tension. Eventually this control can be achieved without feedback from the machine.

The ability to breathe correctly is necessary to attain deep relaxation. However, correct breathing is not as natural or easy as it sounds. Most of us tend to breathe shallowly from our chests, which increases our feelings of tension. All of the relaxation techniques emphasize abdominal breathing in which the abdomen expands during inhalation. Abdominal breathing is an excellent way to elicit the relaxation response and with frequent practice will become second nature to us during our active day.

Relaxation techniques can be learned from books, from experienced practitioners, or from qualified teachers. Biofeedback should be taught by a trained instructor.

Exercise is a method of stress management that is often overlooked. Regular vigorous physical activity will reduce stress levels and impart a feeling of well-being. It can allow us to let go mentally of the stress for a while, at the same time reducing muscle tension.

As we noted in chapter 2, chronic stress can have a detrimental effect on our bodies, psyches, and spirits. Serious medical conditions as well as emotional distress and chronic pain may develop when the stress reaction is allowed to continue. Stress-management techniques interrupt this reaction and result in immediate benefits of a greater sense of well-being and less muscular and emotional tension. They also have a beneficial effect on conditions such as high blood pressure, back pain, headache, dermatitis, and lowered immune response. Incorporating stress management into your daily life helps to prevent such conditions from occurring.

Stress, in and of itself, is not bad. Hans Selye, one of the first stress researchers, called stress "the spice of life." Without stress none of us would get up in the morning, go to work or school, or take care of our families. We must distinguish between stress and challenge. Our goal is not to reduce stress to zero but to improve our ability to cope with it. This quality has been called "hardiness." People who are hardy exhibit the fight-or-flight response to stressors less often than those who are not hardy. Studies show that hardy people have an earnest devotion to themselves, their families, their work, and to larger values. They also feel in control of their lives and view change as a challenge instead of a menace.[19]

Hardy people also use their support network more effectively than those who succumb to stressors. The result is that people who are hardy become ill less often than their overstressed counterparts. Hardiness is an important ingredient in preventing illness and in promoting health. When Bernie Siegel, author of *Love, Medicine, and Miracles*, was asked at a workshop on illness and healing what he recommended we teach our children, he said: "I would teach them that life is full of problems, but you will always overcome them."

INJURY PREVENTION

Case Study

Hilde was a 90-year-old widow in fairly good health who had been living alone since her sister's death. She had poor eyesight and some difficulty in walking. She used a cane and did not get out often. Her house was crowded with furniture, decorative items, and area rugs, which she had collected over the years.

Hilde fell one day in her house, but was able to get up and suffered only a bruise. She had not noticed the edge of a rug and had tripped on it. About a month later, Hilde fell again and this time she broke her hip. She needed surgery and prolonged rehabilitation. She was forced to sell her home.

* * *

Most of us would have called Hilde's mishap an "accident," meaning that the event was random and unpredictable and therefore not preventable. However, it turns out that events like Hilde's fall *are* predictable and preventable. When we examine the statistics, we find that falls are a very common cause of injury among the elderly because of identifiable characteristics found in this age group.

We do not use the word *accident* to describe mishaps that result in injury, but describe the injury according to its cause (e.g., drowning, falls, motor-vehicle-related). We then recommend ways to prevent the injury or to prevent lethal damage if it does occur.

It is estimated that about 75 million Americans are injured every year, resulting in over 150,000 deaths.[20] Injuries are the leading cause of death for persons between the ages of 1 and 45. Motor vehicle collisions account for the greatest number of traumatic injuries and for about 45,000 deaths each year.

Other causes of injury include falls, drowning, fire, electric current, firearms, poisoning, suffocation, and air transportation. The importance of each cause of injury may change depending on age, sex, and race. For instance, suffocation is primarily a problem for children because of their being exposed to plastic bags, getting their heads trapped in tight spaces, and choking on small objects, including certain foods. Falls cause more deaths in the elderly than in any other age group, often because of their impaired mobility and poor vision, unsafe environmental conditions, medications that impair their alertness, and the presence of osteoporosis.

Lethal and nonlethal injuries from firearms are most often intentional. Only about 5 percent are unintentional ("accidental"). Young men between the ages of 15 and 19 have the greatest risk of unintentional death from firearms. However, young black men aged 15 to 24 are most likely to die from homicide. This is the number one health problem in this group. It is possible and often desirable to think of homicide as a public health problem. Viewing all injuries as public health issues helps us think of new methods of prevention.

Knowing who is most likely to sustain an injury because of a certain event helps target those groups for preventive intervention. Traditionally, the prevention of injuries has been in the domain of "accident prevention" programs, which attempt to modify human behavior. This would include education programs to encourage people to buckle their seat belts and to refrain from drinking and driving.

Seat belts can save lives, including yours, even if you are the safest driver around. Seat belts and child safety seats can save your child's life if you are involved in an automobile collision. Protect yourself and your loved ones by using the simple devices that are available to you. We strongly urge you to wear your seat belt every time you ride in a car, starting *now*.

The incidence and severity of injuries can be reduced in other ways. Auto companies could be encouraged to build cars that are less likely to cause injury, with such features as antilock brakes and air bags. These preventive measures work automatically to protect people from injury, and protect those who are least likely to use seat belts (teenagers and drunk drivers).

Preventive interventions for all types of injuries can be based on a simple model developed by Haddon and Baker.[21] This model divides injury prevention into three phases: pre-event, event, and post-event. The event phase is the situation that directly causes the injury. The pre-event phase includes interventions applied before the event occurs, and the post-event phase involves interventions after the injury occurs in order to decrease the likelihood of permanent disability or death.

In the case of motor vehicle crashes, pre-event interventions would include driver education and tough enforcement of drunk driving laws, measures that would make it less likely that the event (the crash) would occur. Interventions in the event phase would include safety features such as padded dashboards, collapsible steering columns, and air bags, which would decrease the likelihood of serious injury during the event. An effective emergency medical system that responds promptly and adequate rehabilitation services for those who are seriously injured are examples of post-event interventions.

By using this model, prevention strategies for all kinds of injuries, both intentional and unintentional, can be developed. Many of these strategies have already been utilized. We now put childproof caps on medicine containers rather than expecting adults to keep medications out of the child's reach, sand is used as a surface in playgrounds to lessen the likelihood of injury, and trauma centers have been developed to treat those with serious injury.

This model of injury prevention provides a framework for thinking about how to prevent injuries in personal life and in the community. For more information, contact the Insurance Institute for Highway Safety in Washington, DC, or the Injury Prevention Center at The Johns Hopkins School of Hygiene and Public Health in Baltimore, Maryland. Another excellent resource is the publication *Injury Prevention: Meeting the Challenge.*[22]

*   *   *

By taking steps to promote our own health, we "turn the corner" from neutral living toward wholeness. These health promotion actions include regular exercise, not smoking, the responsible use of alcohol and medications, avoidance of addictive drugs, positive stress management, and the development of injury-prevention strategies. Another critical area of health behavior is the prevention of specific diseases, which is discussed in chapter 7.

7

Disease Prevention

Preventing illness is obviously better than treating it. Effective prevention avoids the suffering, inconvenience, and cost of illness. The problem is that when we prevent something from happening we cannot prove that our action was the cause of the desired effect. Did stopping smoking keep me from having a heart attack, or would I not have had one anyway?

It is possible, however, when examining groups of people to compare interventions and to look at differences in outcome. If we are interested in finding out whether lowering elevated cholesterol will prevent heart attacks, then we can compare two groups of people with high cholesterol levels. They will be similar in most ways (sex, age, health habits) except that the members of one group will lower their dietary fat intake and the members of the other group will eat normally. If the group that ate less fat shows lower cholesterol levels and fewer heart attacks, and if this result is repeated in other studies, we can conclude that lowering elevated serum cholesterol levels will prevent heart attacks.

Recommendations are developed in disease prevention by doing a number of studies on large groups of people to detect significant trends. By this means, researchers are able to discover *risk factors* for diseases. A risk factor is a characteristic or condition that increases the likelihood that a certain disease or condition will occur. For instance, obesity is a risk factor for diabetes and being a young man is a risk factor for a motor-vehicle-related injury. Some risk factors cannot be changed, such as age, sex, race, and family history. But others are modifiable, such as diet, exercise, and smoking. Our emphasis is on the modifiable risk factors.

Preventive health services are designated primary or secondary. Primary prevention includes interventions intended to keep certain diseases and injuries from happening at all, for example, setting the water heater temperature to no more than 125 degrees F. to prevent scalds. Secondary prevention, or early detection as it is sometimes called, is used to find disease in its early, treatable stage. We use secondary prevention in breast cancer detection, where finding the tumor when it is small improves the chances of cure.

In this chapter we make general recommendations for healthy people. This information should be used as a starting point to find out what you can do to stay healthy. Since each of us is a unique individual, you should rely on your health-care providers to give you directions that are specific to your situation.

HEART DISEASE PREVENTION

Case Study
When Greg came to St. Luke Health Center for a checkup, he was 27-years old and had been healthy all his life. Although he knew he should exercise regularly he found it hard to fit exercise into his schedule as a high school teacher. He was also at increased risk of heart disease because his father had died of a heart attack at age 60.

As expected, Greg's physical exam was entirely normal, but his serum cholesterol level turned out to be high. He was alarmed and became motivated to lower his cholesterol. He made changes in his diet and was able to bring the cholesterol level down to a safe range. He also urged his younger brother to get his cholesterol checked since elevations can run in families. His brother had the test done and found that his cholesterol was also elevated.

Over half-a-million people die from heart attacks every year in this country, and about one million others suffer nonfatal heart attacks. Millions more have chest pain for which they must take medication. Cardiovascular disease is the leading cause of death in the United States. But the good news is that deaths caused by coronary heart disease have been declining significantly since 1968 because of improvements in personal health habits and medical care.

The heart is a muscle that is stimulated by an electrical system to pump blood into the arteries in a rhythmic fashion. The heart needs oxygen to work. Oxygen is carried in the blood that is supplied to the heart via arteries that originate at the base of the aorta and encircle the heart, called the coronary arteries.

All arteries in the body, including the coronary arteries, may be affected by atherosclerosis, an abnormal process that damages the lining of the arteries and causes a thick plaque to build up, obstructing blood flow. If one or more of the coronary arteries becomes narrowed by atherosclerosis, the heart cannot receive adequate oxygen when it is stressed, for instance during exercise. But the heart must continue to pump to keep the person alive. This discrepancy between the supply and demand of oxygen usually causes chest pain (angina pectoris). If the narrowed coronary artery becomes blocked by a clot broken off from an atherosclerotic plaque, no oxygen reaches the area and the heart muscle starts to die. This usually results in severe, unremitting chest pain and is what is known as a myocardial infarction or heart attack.

The infarction can cause the heart to stop beating altogether or to beat too rapidly to pump blood. This can happen within minutes or hours or days. If no emergency medical care is available, it will lead to death. If a large portion of the heart muscle has died it may be unable to pump enough blood to keep the individual alive.

A number of risk factors have been associated with coronary heart disease. High serum cholesterol has been shown to have a direct effect on atherosclerosis. How other factors, such as lack of exercise, contribute to heart disease is not clear. Nevertheless, studies of populations have shown that the presence of certain factors increases a person's risk of having a heart attack. The nonmodifiable risk factors for coronary heart disease are age, male sex, and family history. The modifiable risk factors strongly associated with heart disease are cigarette smoking, elevated serum cholesterol, elevated blood pressure, and diabetes. Other risk factors that have a weaker relationship but probably contribute to heart disease are physical inactivity, Type A behavior, and obesity.

Cigarette smoke increases total serum cholesterol and LDL cholesterol (the "bad" kind) and decreases HDL cholesterol (the "good" kind). These conditions promote atherosclerosis. Besides its role in atherosclerosis, cigarette smoking increases the amount of carbon monoxide in the blood, which makes it harder for the blood to carry oxygen. The nicotine in cigarettes increases the heart rate, which raises the demand for oxygen. The decreased supply coupled with an increased demand for oxygen puts a strain on the heart.

Cigarette smoking doubles the risk of having a heart attack. If every smoker quit smoking, the incidence of coronary heart disease would plummet. Smokers who quit lower their risk of heart attack immediately, and their risk of heart attack approaches that of the non-smoker's within 10 years. (For a further discussion of smoking cessation, see chapter 6.)

The heart pumps blood into an arterial system composed of vessels of decreasing size. Blood passes from arteries to arterioles to capillaries. At the capillary level, the nutrients are delivered to the cells and waste products are picked up. The blood then travels back to the lungs and heart through the venous system. The arterioles can be compared to the nozzle on a hose. In a hose, water flows from a source and meets a certain amount of resistance at the nozzle. The degree of resistance is controlled by the opening in the nozzle; the smaller the opening, the greater is the pressure within the hose. Likewise, the arterioles control how much pressure is present in the arteries by constricting and enlarging. This process is influenced by many variables, including blood volume, hormones, and stress.

Pressure in the arteries is measured in millimeters of mercury using a blood pressure cuff and stethoscope. The reading is given in two numbers separated by a slash, for instance, 116/72. The upper number represents the pressure in the artery (usually in the arm) when the heart is pumping blood (systole), called the systolic blood pressure. The lower number is the pressure in the artery when the heart is relaxing (diastole), or the diastolic blood pressure. An average systolic reading of 140 or more and/or an average diastolic reading of 90 or more measured at least twice on two or more occasions is classified as high blood pressure or hypertension. (See Table 7-1.)

Approximately 58 million Americans have elevated blood pressure or are taking medication for it.[1] The higher the blood pressure the greater is the risk of heart disease and stroke.

Hypertension rarely causes symptoms. That is why it is important to have a blood-pressure check at least every two years if it is normal. If it is not normal, follow your doctor's instructions on how often to have it checked. A single high reading does not mean hypertension. It must be elevated on at least two occasions.

High blood pressure can be brought down in a number of ways. The following recommendations are based on the National Institutes of Health report on *The Detection, Evaluation, and Treatment of High Blood Pressure.*[2] As discussed in chapter 5, sodium restriction is often effective in lowering blood pressure. This doesn't work for everyone, but it is impossible to tell in advance who will benefit, so all hypertensives should limit their salt intake to four to six grams a day. Increasing dietary potassium and/or calcium may also help to lower

TABLE 7-1.

Classification of Blood Pressure in Adults Age 18 Years or Older[a]

Range, mm Hg	Category[b]
Diastolic	
<85	Normal blood pressure
85–89	High normal blood pressure
90–104	Mild hypertension
105–114	Moderate hypertension
≥115	Severe hypertension
Systolic, when diastolic blood pressure is <90	
<140	Normal blood pressure
140–159	Borderline isolated systolic hypertension
≥160	Isolated systolic hypertension

[a]Classification based on the average of two or more readings on two or more occasions

[b]A classification of borderline isolated systolic hypertension (SBP 140 to 159) or isolated systolic hypertension (SBP ≥160) takes precedence over high normal blood pressure (DBP 85–89) when both occur in the same person. High normal blood pressure (DBP 85–89) takes precedence over a classification of normal blood pressure (SBP <140) when both occur in the same person.

Source: Department of Health and Human Services, *The 1988 Report of the Joint National Committee on Detection, Evaluation, and Treatment of High Blood Pressure*, prepared by National High Blood Pressure Education Program, National Institutes of Health, NIH Pub. No. 88-1088 (Washington, DC, 1988).

blood pressure, but check with your doctor before taking supplements of these elements, especially if you have kidney disease or are taking blood pressure medication.

Body weight and blood pressure are related. If an obese hypertensive person loses weight, the blood pressure will often decrease. An effective way to achieve weight loss is by aerobic exercise, since that alone will help lower blood pressure. However, if you have high blood pressure and want to start an exercise program, see your doctor first.

Some people's blood pressure is very sensitive to alcohol consumption. In those cases, alcohol should be restricted to less than 2 ounces of whiskey, 8 ounces of wine, or 24 ounces of beer a day, or eliminated altogether.

Smoking causes a short-term elevation of blood pressure but has not been associated with hypertension. Smoking may, however, interfere with other treatments intended to reduce risk for heart disease.

Biofeedback and relaxation procedures have been used effectively for lowering elevated blood pressure. Psychologist James Lynch has successfully taught hypertensive individuals how to control their blood pressure by learning to communicate differently. He measures blood pressure during psychotherapy sessions to illustrate to the client the relationship between speaking and blood pressure elevation.[3]

For mild hypertension, some or all of these nonpharmacologic (non-drug) treatments can be tried. They will sometimes be all that is needed. Medications for hypertension are used for people whose blood pressure does not respond adequately to other methods. The nonpharmacologic approaches should be continued even if the individual is taking medication since they may reduce the dose necessary to control the blood pressure.

It would be prudent even for people with normal blood pressure to follow these recommendations, especially those with a family history of hypertension, high normal blood pressure readings, and African ancestry. In doing so, they may be able to avoid hypertension and its adverse health effects.[4]

Cholesterol is a fatlike substance (lipid) that is a necessary component in all of our cells. It is also needed to make sex hormones. Our bodies can manufacture all the cholesterol we need, but if we eat animal products, including eggs and milk, we also get cholesterol in our diets. Cholesterol travels in the bloodstream in little packages called lipoproteins. The level of cholesterol in the blood is determined by genetic inheritance, diet, weight, and physical activity.

Total serum cholesterol is measured by determining the level of cholesterol present in the lipoprotein packages. There are three categories of lipoproteins: VLDL or very low-density, LDL or low-density, and HDL or high-density lipoproteins. Most of the cholesterol is in the LDL portion, which is the type associated with atherosclerosis. HDL actually helps rid the body of cholesterol, and a high level of this lipoprotein is beneficial.

Elevated serum cholesterol is associated with an increased risk of coronary heart disease. Lowering total and LDL-cholesterol will reduce that risk. The recommendations that follow are based on the

1988 report from the National Cholesterol Education Program sponsored by the National Heart, Lung, and Blood Institute.[5]

If you have not had your cholesterol checked, do it this year. If your cholesterol level is in the desirable range, have the test done at least every five years. A level over 200 but below 240 mg/dl falls into the borderline-high category. Anything at or above 240 is considered a high total cholesterol level. Table 7-2 shows the risk categories and recommended follow-up.

If a screening test is done for cholesterol and the level is over 200,

TABLE 7-2.

Initial Classification and Recommended Follow-up Based on Total Cholesterol

A. Classification

<200 mg/dl	Desirable blood cholesterol
200-239 mg/dl	Borderline-high blood cholesterol
≥240 mg/dl	High blood cholesterol

B. Recommended Follow-up

Total cholesterol <200 mg/dl	Repeat within five years
Total cholesterol 200-239 mg/dl *Without* definite CHD or two other CHD risk factors (one of which can be male sex)[a]	Dietary information and recheck annually
With definite CHD or two other CHD risk factors (one of which can be male sex)[a]	Lipoprotein analysis; further action based on LDL-cholesterol level
Total cholesterol ≥240	

[a]CHD (Coronary Heart Disease) risk factors: male sex, family history of premature CHD, smoking, hypertension, low HDL, diabetes, definite cerebrovascular or peripheral vascular disease, or severe obesity.

Source: Department of Health and Human Services, *Report of the Expert Panel on Detection, Evaluation, and Treatment of High Blood Cholesterol in Adults*, prepared by National Cholesterol Education Program, National Institutes of Health, NIH Pub. No. 88-2925 (Washington, DC, 1988).

the test should be repeated. Your physician can tell you which category you fall into and what kind of treatment you need.

The mainstay of treatment for high cholesterol is diet. If your serum cholesterol is elevated you will probably be advised to decrease your total intake of fat, especially animal fat. Most fats in the diet should be of the polyunsaturated and monounsaturated variety (see chapter 5). Poultry without skin and fish are very good low-fat sources of protein that can be substituted for high-fat red meats and cheeses. In fact, eating fish that contain omega-3 fatty acids, which live in deep, cold ocean waters, may protect against heart disease. These fish include halibut, herring, salmon, tuna, sardines, and others. It's helpful also to eat oat products and beans, since the fiber in these foods has been found to lower cholesterol. These changes should not be temporary but rather lifelong habits.

If you are overweight, weight reduction may lower LDL and raise HDL levels. Exercise may also help to increase HDL-cholesterol.

Recommended dietary changes are shown in Table 7-3.

Reduction of saturated fat to 10 percent of total calories will usually lower serum cholesterol to a safe range. Sometimes, however, serum cholesterol does not decrease enough and more changes must be made. Your physician should monitor your serum cholesterol and advise you if your intake of cholesterol and saturated fat needs to be lowered even further. In a small number of cases even this degree of fat restriction is not enough and a cholesterol-lowering drug must be used in addition.

The low-fat diets that are generally recommended are palatable and enjoyable, but if you are used to eating a lot of fatty meat, cream sauces, cheese, and pastries, it may take some time to get used to the change. However, most people are able to adapt and even enjoy the new tastes of lower-fat foods.

People who are diabetic, especially women past menopause, are at increased risk of developing heart disease.[6] Even those women who are not diagnosed as diabetic but who have a milder, usually unrecognized, form of the disease (glucose intolerance), are more likely to develop coronary heart disease. Diabetics often have elevated cholesterol levels and are more predisposed to developing atherosclerosis.[7] Reduction of the risk of heart disease for diabetics is best done by weight control and exercise, which will also help control blood sugar.

Obesity makes it more likely that a person will develop high blood pressure, high cholesterol, or diabetes, three strong risk factors for coronary heart disease.[8] Overweight as a direct risk factor for heart

TABLE 7-3.

Recommended Diet Modifications to Lower Blood Cholesterol

	Choose	*Decrease*
Fish, chicken, turkey, and lean meats	Fish, poultry without skin, lean cuts of beef, lamb, pork or veal, shellfish	Fatty cuts of beef, lamb, pork; spareribs, organ meats, regular cold cuts, sausage, hotdogs, bacon, sardines, roe
Skim and low-fat milk, cheese, yogurt, and dairy substitutes	Skim or 1 percent fat milk, buttermilk	Whole milk (4 percent fat); cream, half and half, 2 percent milk, imitation milk products, most non-dairy creamers, whipped toppings
	Nonfat and low-fat yogurt	Whole-milk yogurt
	Low-fat cottage cheese	Whole-milk cottage cheese
	Low-fat cheeses, farmer or pot cheeses	All natural cheeses
		Low-fat or "light" cream cheese and sour cream; cream cheese, sour cream
	Sherbet, sorbet	Ice cream
Eggs	Egg whites (2 whites = 1 whole egg in recipes), cholesterol-free substitutes	Egg yolks
Fruits and vegetables	Fresh, frozen, canned, or dried	Vegetables prepared in butter, cream, or other sauces

TABLE 7-3.

Recommended Diet Modifications to Lower Blood Cholesterol

	Choose	Decrease
Breads and cereals	Homemade baked goods using unsaturated oils sparingly, angel food cake, low-fat crackers, and cookies	Commercial baked goods: pies, cakes, doughnuts, croissants, pastries, muffins, biscuits, high-fat crackers and cookies
	Rice, pasta	Egg noodles
	Whole-grain breads and cereals	Breads in which eggs are major ingredient
Fats and oils	Baking cocoa	Chocolate
	Unsaturated vegetable oils	Butter, coconut oil, palm oil, palm kernel oil, lard, bacon fat
	Margarine or shortening made from one of the unsaturated oils, diet margarine	
	Mayonnaise, salad dressings made with unsaturated oils; low-fat dressings	Dressings made with egg yolk
	Seeds and nuts	Coconut

Source: Department of Health and Human Services, Report of the Expert Panel on Detection, Evaluation, and Treatment of High Blood Cholesterol in Adults, prepared by National Cholesterol Education Program, National Institutes of Health, NIH Pub. No. 88-2925 (Washington, DC, 1988).

disease has been more difficult to prove. However, weight loss, with or without exercise, probably reduces the likelihood that an individual will develop heart disease.[9]

Evidence is accumulating that physical activity, especially aerobic exercise, helps lower the risk of heart disease. This is not only because of its beneficial effects on blood pressure, cholesterol, and weight but also because of some direct influence on cardiovascular function. There is a small risk of sudden death during strenuous exercise, but it is outweighed by the long-term benefits to health and well-being. The principles of good exercise programs were outlined in chapter 6.

In the 1970s cardiologists Friedman and Rosenman published studies on the relationship between behavior and heart disease. They found that a constellation of behavioral characteristics they called Type A was associated with a greater risk of heart disease. Those who did not exhibit the characteristics were not at increased risk and were called Type B. Traits of a Type A person are a sense of time urgency, excessive competitiveness, concern with quantity rather than quality, an inability to relax without feeling guilty, doing more than one thing at a time, and impatience.[10] People with Type B behavior, on the other hand, value the content rather than the number of their accomplishments, take time to enjoy and dream, are less hostile and competitive, and are more accepting of themselves and others.

Friedman and Rosenman believe it is possible to alter a person's behavior from Type A to Type B, and in so doing, to lessen the likelihood of heart attack. Type A behavior is rewarded in our society, often with money and prestige. However, it is often the less-competitive Type B persons who are more productive because of their ability to deal effectively with stressful situations.

Other researchers have found that the Type A-Type B categories are not precise enough predictors for coronary heart disease. Dr. Robert Eliot believes that it is not a person's actions that predispose to heart attack but rather the internal physiologic reactions to stressful events.[11] He calls people who have elevated blood pressure and lowered cardiac output during competitive activity or mental stress "hot reactors." Many of them appear on the outside to be Type B individuals, but they have a similar risk for heart disease as people who are Type A. Dr. Eliot believes it is necessary to help hot reactors alter their responses to stress in order to avoid a heart attack.

Behavior change is not easy to accomplish, but it can be facilitated through the stress-management techniques we described in chapter 6. A person's behavior reflects his or her attitude about life. We act according to our feelings about our own worth and that of others, the accomplishments and activities we value, how we like to spend leisure time, and what we find humorous. As Dr. Friedman has said, it may be important to know the yield of peaches in an orchard, but we would be missing a lot if we didn't also appreciate the beauty of the peach blossoms.

CANCER PREVENTION

One out of every three of us will develop cancer in his or her lifetime. Although billions of dollars have been spent on cancer treatment and research, over 400,000 people die every year in this country from cancer. In fact, few strides have been made in the treatment of the more common cancers.[12] Fortunately, there is now a growing interest in what can be done to prevent cancer from occurring in the first place.

Researchers estimate that more than 90 percent of cancer is caused by "environmental" factors.[13] These include not only carcinogens in our air, water, and food but also life-style behaviors, such as diet and smoking. The remaining 10 (or more) percent is the result of hereditary causes not under our control. This is good news; there may be a lot we can do individually and collectively to avoid cancer.

Cancer is the uncontrolled growth and dispersal of cells. A number of different types of cancer can arise in almost any tissue in the body; however, it is thought that cancer actually develops by the same process in each instance. The transformation of a normal cell into a cancerous one is believed to be a two-step process. The first step is called *initiation* and is thought to be rapid and irreversible. It is characterized by damage to the cell's DNA (genetic code) by chemical or physical agents. The second step, called *promotion,* is, in contrast, slow and somewhat reversible. The result is a cell that is more extensively transformed into an abnormal one. The two steps are necessary for cancer to develop. Initiation must precede promotion, but there is no definite time interval between the two stages. Promotion may immediately follow initiation or years may elapse between the two events. Usually initiation and promotion are caused by different agents, but not always.

The primary prevention of cancer is possible if we make changes in our tobacco use, diet, and radiation exposure. (Occupational and environmental hazards are discussed later in this chapter.) If you don't smoke, don't start. If you do smoke you will greatly reduce the risk of cancer by stopping now. You will diminish the risk not only of lung cancer but also of cancer of the mouth, esophagus, larynx, bladder, pancreas, and cervix. Lung cancer alone causes almost 90,000 deaths a year in the United States. It accounts for about 20 percent of all cancer, and about 85 percent of lung cancer in men is attributable to smoking.[14] Lung cancer is usually diagnosed late, so its prognosis is often grim. Cigarette smoke contains both initiators and promoters of cancer, and it is even more deadly in the presence of certain occupational and environmental hazards, such as asbestos and radon.[15] No amount of day-to-day environmental pollution can compare to the burden of carcinogens put into the body if you smoke. (See chapter 6 on smoking cessation.)

Tobacco use other than cigarette smoking also increases the risk of cancer. Cigar and pipe smoking are risk factors for cancer of the lung, larynx, esophagus, mouth, and throat. Pipe smoking also increases the likelihood of developing lip cancer. Smokeless tobacco (chewing tobacco and snuff) can cause mouth cancer.

Specific cancers occur at different rates in different areas of the world. For instance, stomach cancer is common in Japan but is declining in the United States. At the same time, colon cancer and breast cancer are important causes of death in this country but are less frequent in Japan. We might attribute these differences to genetics, but a number of studies have shown that they may be related to diet. Descendants of Japanese who immigrate to Hawaii have higher rates of colon and breast cancer than their parents. Grandchildren of Japanese who move to the United States mainland have rates similar to our national rates. So life-style factors, including diet, must play a role in the development of cancer.

It appears that some carcinogens, including those found in food, can cause an oxidation reaction in cells. This is the same sort of reaction that occurs when fat becomes rancid on exposure to air. The products of this reaction are called *free radicals*, which are highly energized, unstable compounds. In order to regain their stability these compounds must discharge their extra energy. Normally, our bodies can handle a certain amount of free radicals, but if the burden is too great the detoxification process may be overwhelmed. The result of this damage may be the initiation or promotion of cancer.[16]

A variety of dietary components and additives capable of causing an oxidation reaction are suspected of being initiators of cancer. Some are put on food, pesticides, for example, or in food to preserve it, such as nitrites in processed or cured meats. Other carcinogens are found naturally in certain foods, such as mushrooms, alfalfa sprouts, and black pepper, or may contaminate diseased or damaged food, such as grains, peanuts, and fruit. Some foods become potential initiators of cancer when they are processed or exposed to air, such as rancid fats, or when they are cooked by frying or charcoal broiling.

Foods that are highly processed by heating, powdering, and irradiating may also become initiators.[17]

The good news is that foods also contain nutrients that may protect us against cancer. Some of these components are antioxidants, that is, compounds that detoxify the free radicals produced by oxidative reactions. They include vitamin C, vitamin E, carotene, and the mineral selenium. Research has shown that the consumption of vitamin C-rich foods is associated with a lower risk of cancer of the stomach and esophagus,[18] possibly because of the ability of vitamin C to block the formation of cancer-causing nitrosamines from nitrates and nitrites found in food and water. Nitrates and nitrites are turned into nitrosamines by bacteria present in the digestive tract. Nitrates in water come from fertilizer runoff, and they are found naturally in some vegetables, such as beets, celery, and radishes. Nitrites are added to some meat, fish, beer, and dairy products. Vitamin C is present in citrus fruits, strawberries, papaya, potatoes, dark green leafy vegetables, and broccoli.

Vitamin E is an antioxidant and prevents the formation of nitrosamines. Also, since it is fat-soluble it has a role in limiting the creation of free radicals in fats and oils. Vitamin E is found in rolled oats and wheat germ, polyunsaturated oils (especially wheat germ oil), and seeds and nuts. There is no convincing evidence that vitamin E can protect against cancer, but a few studies show some protective effect for lung and breast cancer.[19]

Selenium, another antioxidant, is a mineral that is required in minute amounts in humans. It is found in lean meats and organ meats, seafood, whole-grain products, milk, and many vegetables. The actual selenium level in these foods is difficult to predict, however, because it depends on the level in the soil, which varies widely from one region to the next. This makes it hard to determine the association of selenium intake and cancer. Some studies show a relationship between cancer and low serum selenium.[20] The conclusions are further complicated by the possibility that selenium may be most effective in conjunction with vitamin A and/or vitamin E.[21]

Carotene, a precursor of vitamin A, is found in dark green and yellow vegetables and acts as an antioxidant. Vitamin A, which is found preformed only in animal products, controls the ability of cells to take on specific functions and characteristics, called *differentiation*. A basic feature of cancer is a loss of cell differentiation. So it makes sense that vitamin A and carotenoids such as beta-carotene might have a role in cancer prevention. Studies have shown a protective effect of beta-carotene against lung cancer in humans.[22]

These inconclusive results make it difficult to decide whether or not to use supplements for protection against cancer. However, it is safe to recommend eating more of those foods with vitamins A, C, and E, selenium, and beta-carotene (see Table 7-4). If you want to take supplements, we recommend that you consult a qualified physician or nutritionist, since vitamin A and selenium can be dangerous in large amounts.

TABLE 7-4.

Food Choices That May Help Prevent Cancer

- Eat foods with vitamin C, such as oranges, grapefruit, strawberries, cantaloupe, mango, papaya, green pepper, spinach, broccoli, brussels sprouts, cabbage, cauliflower, kale, and turnip greens.
- Increase intake of vitamin E by eating wheat germ and rolled oats and by using unsaturated oils such as corn, peanut, safflower, sunflower, and wheat germ. Nuts and seeds also have vitamin E but are high in fat so should be used sparingly.
- Choose foods with selenium, such as seafood and whole grains.
- Eat foods rich in beta-carotene, such as carrots, butternut squash, sweet potato, cantaloupe, greens, kale, bok choy, broccoli, apricots, spinach, and acorn squash.
- Choose more low-fat and fewer high-fat foods. (See Table 7-3)
- Increase fiber intake by choosing whole-grain breads, cereals, and pastas; dried beans and peas; fruits and vegetables; and nuts and seeds.
- Eat vegetables from the cabbage family (cruciferous vegetables): bok choy, broccoli, brussels sprouts, cabbage, cauliflower, collards, kale, kohlrabi, mustard greens, rutabagas, and turnips and their greens.
- Reduce foods with added nitrites and nitrates and charcoal-broiled foods.

Another component of diet that may protect against cancer is fiber. Dietary fiber is that part of plants that humans are unable to digest or digest incompletely. It serves the purpose of helping to move food through the digestive tract. In areas of the world in which fiber intake is high, less colon cancer is seen than in the United States and other industrialized countries. Fiber's role in colon cancer prevention may be the result of its ability to decrease transit time, bind carcinogens, or eliminate fats more efficiently from the digestive tract.[23] This type of insoluble fiber is found in whole grains of all kinds, fruits, vegetables, dry peas, and beans. Americans eat about 11 grams of fiber a day. The National Cancer Institute recommends that this be increased to 20 to 30 grams per day by eating more high-fiber foods.[24] Also, areas with low consumption of cruciferous vegetables (broccoli, kale, cauliflower, cabbage, etc.) have a higher incidence of colon cancer. It is thought that these vegetables may be protective.[25]

A diet high in fat is believed to contribute to the development of cancer, especially cancer of the breast, colon, and prostate. Countries in which the populations have low-fat diets tend to have lower incidences of these cancers. To prevent breast cancer it may be necessary to decrease fat intake to 20 percent of total calories.[26] The average American eats a diet of 40 percent fat. There are no definitive recommendations yet, but women should lower their total dietary fat to no more than 30 percent of total calories, which is consistent with a heart-healthy diet. This modification may also help to prevent other cancers.

Alcohol consumption has been found to be associated with an increased risk of cancer of the esophagus, especially if the individual smokes cigarettes. Heavy consumption of beer is associated with a higher risk of rectal cancer.[27]

Unfortunately, research in the area of diet and cancer is inconclusive, so we cannot make any definitive recommendations. As British researchers Doll and Peto said in 1981 about cancer in the United States: "For many years there has been strong but indirect evidence that most of the cancers that are currently common could be made less so by suitable modification of national dietary practices . . . but there is still no precise and reliable evidence as to exactly what dietary changes would be of major importance."[28] If we wait for definitive evidence we may be allowing a large number of preventable deaths to occur from cancer. The recommendations listed in Table 7-4 are healthful ones and there is some indication that they can help prevent cancer.

Sunlight is a cause of two types of skin cancer, squamous cell and basal cell. These cancers are usually found on exposed parts of the body, more often on light-skinned individuals, and their risk increases with increasing amounts of sun exposure. These types of cancer are not dangerous if they are removed before they invade deeper tissues. They are preventable by avoiding or limiting exposure to the sun. Skin cancer is caused by ultraviolet A radiation that is present during the day. The best protection is to stay in the shade or to wear a hat and clothing that cover your skin. Physical sun blocks, such as zinc oxide, are useful on limited areas of the body, such as the nose and lips. A sunscreen will offer some protection, according to its Sun Protection Factor (SPF). The higher the SPF, through 15, the longer will be the protection. It has been estimated that regular use of sunscreen of SPF 15 during the first 18 years of life decreases the lifetime incidence of these cancers by 78 percent.[29]

A third type of skin cancer is malignant melanoma, which is much more dangerous because it can metastasize and cause death. However, its relation to sun exposure is complex. Melanoma may be associated with episodes of severe sunburn, rather than more regular but less severe exposures.

Other types of radiation can contribute to cancer in humans. Most of this exposure is the result of ionizing radiation, which includes X rays, environmental sources, and nuclear weapon fallout. Medical X rays account for the greatest excess exposure above and beyond background radiation in the environment. In order to minimize diagnostic X rays as a cancer-causing agent, you should avoid unnecessary X rays, make sure to receive the lowest possible dose, and request lead shielding for areas of the body that do not need to be exposed. Only about 1 percent of cancers are thought to be caused by radiation, but many of these cases are preventable if precautions are taken to minimize exposure.[30]

Secondary prevention, or early detection of disease that has already begun, is feasible for a small number of important cancers including cancers of the breast, cervix, colon, and rectum. In these cases procedures are available to find disease at an early stage *and* treatment at this stage results in greater chance of cure. For other types of cancer, such as lung cancer, tests (chest X ray) are available that can detect the tumor before symptoms occur, but this doesn't always improve the chance of cure. In the case of lung cancer, studies have shown that persons who received periodic chest X rays (every 4 to 12 months) had the same death rate from lung cancer as those who had less frequent chest X rays.[31]

Perhaps the most widely used early detection procedure is the Pap smear, named after Dr. George Papanicolaou. Cells are scraped off the cervix onto slides that are examined under a microscope. The technician looks for abnormal cells that are precursors for cancer. Ideally, the Pap smear detects cells in this precancerous state when they can be removed by local surgery or laser treatment. Deaths resulting from cervical cancer have declined markedly in this country probably because of the widespread use of this test. Many women, however, have never had a Pap smear and are at risk of dying from this preventable disease.

Certain viruses may be associated with cervical cancer.[32] Women who have genital herpes infection are at greater risk of cancer of the cervix. Women who have genital warts or are infected with the virus that causes the warts (papilloma virus) also have an increased risk. Pap smears do not detect these infections, and special tests must be done to see if the viruses are present.[33]

All women who are or have been sexually active should get a Pap smear every one to three years. Testing should begin at the age when sexual intercourse is initiated and may be discontinued at age 65 if there is a documented history of consistently normal Pap smears.[34] If there is a history of cervical abnormalities, sexually transmitted diseases, multiple sexual partners, or early onset of sexual intercourse, the test should be done at more frequent intervals. A health-care provider can suggest the best schedule for individual situations.

Breast cancer is the most common cancer among women, affecting about 1 in 10 in the United States. There are many risk factors for breast cancer, most of them not modifiable. Risk for the disease increases with age and increases also if the woman is white, affluent, and unmarried. Occurrence of breast cancer in a woman's mother or sister is a significant risk factor. Women whose menstrual periods began at an early age and who have a late menopause also are at greater jeopardy, as are women who have never had children or who had their first child after the age of 30. (Conversely, women who have their ovaries removed before reaching menopause are at lower risk.) A history of fibrocystic disease seems to increase the risk for developing breast cancer.[35]

Modifiable risk factors for this disease probably have less influence on its development. They include a high-fat diet, obesity in postmenopausal women, and *high* doses of radiation.[36] The role of oral estrogen, both in contraceptive pills and for the prevention of osteoporosis, is not at all clear.

The *primary* prevention of breast cancer is difficult because of nonmodifiable risk factors. Therefore emphasis has been put on early detection of tumors. This is done by means of three complementary methods: breast self-exam, examination by a health-care professional, and mammography.

Breast self-exam (BSE) should be started when women are 18 years old and should be done once a month for the rest of their lives. Most women don't do it; some say that they don't know what they are looking for. The point is to feel if there has been a change from the previous months. A lump needs to be checked by a doctor. Sometimes physicians find lumps, but more often it is the woman who discovers it, so the annual exam cannot be depended upon as the only preventive procedure. BSE instructions can be obtained from the American Cancer Society, but it is best to learn directly from a health-care provider.

Routine mammography as a screening procedure has been shown to reduce the death rate from breast cancer for women age 50 and above.[37] A mammogram is a low-dose X ray of the breast that can detect most tumors. It can detect lumps that are too small to be felt. At this early stage, the cancer cells usually have not spread to the lymph nodes, so the cancer is curable in about 90 percent of the cases. Mammograms, however, do not detect all lumps, even cancerous ones, so it is still important to do BSE and have annual exams. The US Preventive Services Task Force, experts who make recommendations to primary care providers about preventive services, has proposed the following interventions for breast cancer in women without symptoms: annual clinical breast exam (CBE) by a health-care professional for women age 40 to 49 and annual CBE and mammogram for women age 50 to about 75.[38] For women whose mother or sister developed premenopausal breast cancer, regular CBE and mammography should start as early as age 35. The American Cancer Society, the American Medical Association, and a number of physician specialty organizations suggest that mammography start at age 40 or earlier for all women. However, this recommendation is based on the results of only one scientific study.[39] If you have any questions about when to start having CBE and mammograms, see your doctor.

Cancer of the colon and rectum (also called colorectal cancer) is the second most common type of cancer in the United States. Many researchers believe that it can be prevented through diet, but there is no definitive proof. Emphasis for prevention of colorectal cancer has been mainly on early detection.

Three screening procedures are available for the detection of a tumor of the lower gastrointestinal tract. The least invasive test is to check the stool for blood. Many, though not all, cancers of the GI tract bleed, which produces a positive test. However, noncancerous conditions in the stomach and intestines can also cause bleeding, making the test falsely positive for cancer. Then the individual will have to undergo a more invasive procedure to see why bleeding is occurring. This procedure involves a direct examination of the colon with a flexible tube and light (colonoscopy). If suspicious growths, such as polyps, are found they can be biopsied.

A second screening test is the rectal exam. This procedure will find tumors in the lower part of the rectum only and these account for a small proportion of all colorectal cancers.

A third procedure involves looking at the rectum and lower portion of the colon with a tube (sigmoidoscopy). As with colonoscopy, biopsies can be done, but this procedure does not examine a large portion of the colon in which tumors may arise.

Unfortunately, none of these screening tests has been shown to be effective in reducing mortality in asymptomatic patients with colorectal cancer.[40] Currently, studies are being done to determine the effectiveness of fecal occult blood testing and sigmoidoscopy as screening tests. Until the results of these studies are in, the US Preventive Services Task Force recommends that those who have been getting fecal occult blood testing and/or sigmoidoscopy done should continue the screening. But for those who have not received these tests there are insufficient grounds for initiating them at this point. However, for those 50 years of age or older who have a risk factor for colorectal cancer (immediate relative with colorectal cancer; personal history of uterine, ovarian, or breast cancer; or previous history of inflammatory bowel disease, adenomatous polyps, or colorectal cancer), it may be prudent to have these tests done on a regular basis.[41] If you are not sure whether you fit into a high-risk category, talk to your doctor.

AIDS PREVENTION

AIDS is a preventable disease. We know how the virus is transmitted and how best to avoid it. AIDS prevention requires effort by the public health community as well as the individual. Individuals need accurate information and the opportunity to ask questions and express fears. Health agencies, public and private, need to provide information and allay fears. Until a vaccine is developed, however, the responsibility for ending the spread of the disease rests with each individual.

A-I-D-S stand for Acquired Immune Deficiency Syndrome. It is "acquired" because it is not a hereditary condition. "Immune deficiency" means that the immune system is not working to defend the body from infections and cancer. "Syndrome" indicates that AIDS is diagnosed by the presence of certain types of diseases (not specific symptoms), of which only some are present at any one time. The information that follows is based on the *Surgeon General's Report on Acquired Immune Deficiency Syndrome*,[42] unless otherwise noted.

AIDS was first described in 1981 as a syndrome affecting homosexual men. We have since learned that anyone can get it. AIDS is transmitted by a virus known as HIV, or Human Immunodeficiency Virus. Once it enters the bloodstream, the HIV is able to infect special cells of the immune system, known as T4 lymphocytes, which play a central role in protection against foreign organisms and cancer cells. Although antibodies are produced when the infection occurs, they are not effective in ridding the body of the virus. The AIDS virus is able to infect other cells of the immune system, macrophages and monocytes, that travel all over the body. The virus hides in these cells and may infect various parts of the body, including the brain.

Because the immune system is weakened, a person with AIDS is more vulnerable to "opportunistic infections," diseases that take advantage of the body's lowered resistance. Some of the more common of these diseases are *Pneumocystis carinii* pneumonia, Kaposi's sarcoma (a type of cancer), tuberculosis, Candida, and other infections and cancers. The virus can infect brain cells directly and cause dementia and blindness. A person dying of AIDS may appear emaciated and wasted because of weight loss, diarrhea, vomiting, and lack of appetite.

The syndrome itself is often preceded by a less severe form of HIV infection called AIDS-Related Complex, or ARC. People with this syndrome have nonspecific symptoms that are similar to a bad case of mononucleosis: fatigue, weight loss, diarrhea, swollen glands, fever, and nightsweats. People with ARC often develop AIDS.

In a third form of infection with HIV, the individual has no symptoms at all. It is estimated that one and a half million Americans are infected with the AIDS virus but are not sick. About 20 to 30 percent of those infected with HIV develop AIDS in five years.[43] This incubation period, the time from infection to illness, may be much longer in others. During this time the virus is present in the immune system but does not cause a breakdown of immune defenses. It is not clear why some people are able to resist the damaging effects of the virus longer than others. This is probably the most dangerous form of HIV infection regarding transmission, since the infected person may be unaware that he or she is carrying the virus.

The only way to find out if an individual has been exposed is by having an HIV antibody test done. This blood test does not check for the presence of the virus itself but looks for antibodies to the virus.

If the antibodies are present in repeated tests, the test is positive for HIV. This means there has been exposure to the virus. It does not indicate AIDS since AIDS is a diagnosis made by the presence of certain diseases in conjunction with a positive test for HIV. Unfortunately, it can take six weeks to six months or sometimes longer for the antibodies to be formed once a person has contracted the virus. During the first few weeks after exposure a person can have the AIDS virus and be capable of passing the virus on to someone else, but the HIV antibody test will be negative. So if there is a possibility of exposure, the test should be done no earlier than six weeks after suspected contact. If the test is negative, it would be best to have it repeated five or six months later.

The virus is transmitted from one person to another in essentially two ways: sexual relations and blood. Not only homosexual men are at risk of contracting the AIDS virus through sex. Heterosexuals are in jeopardy if they have vaginal or anal intercourse with an infected person. Oral-genital sex is probably risky too. The more sexual partners one has, the greater is the risk of getting AIDS. It is especially risky to have sex with prostitutes or with someone who uses intravenous drugs.

The safest sexual behavior is to have one uninfected partner who has no other partners, or to practice abstinence. If one partner is infected, or if it is uncertain and intercourse is desired, then a condom should be used. Latex condoms offer the greatest protection (rather than natural ones or "skins"), but they are not 100 percent effective. They can leak or break, and they have to be used correctly each time. A small amount of semen may come out of the penis before ejaculation, so the condom must be put on at the beginning of an erection, and the semen cannot be allowed to leak around the condom when the penis is withdrawn after intercourse. For heterosexual intercourse, women are advised to use spermicide, since the spermicide may also kill the AIDS virus. If a lubricant is used, it should be a water-based one (not petroleum jelly, cream, or oil, which may damage the condom).

Exposure to infected blood is the second major way that the AIDS virus is transmitted. In the United States this happens most often through the sharing of used needles for illicit drug use. After a person injects drugs, a small amount of blood is left in the needle and syringe. If the blood is infected with HIV and another person uses that needle and syringe, then the second person is exposed to the virus. Even the smallest amount of blood left in a needle or syringe can contain the live virus and put the user at risk. The best advice is not to use

intravenous drugs. Drug users who cannot get into a treatment program should use clean needles and syringes each time or disinfect
them with bleach. (One part bleach diluted in 10 parts water will kill
the AIDS virus.)

Before March 1985 there was no good screening test for antibody
to HIV and some people became infected through blood transfusions.
Now there is a reliable test, and all blood is screened before it is used
and contaminated blood is thrown out. Infected blood may pass
through if it was donated before antibodies to the virus have developed; however, since persons who have engaged in risky behaviors
are discouraged from donating blood, this is estimated to happen
very infrequently.

People with hemophilia often receive blood products that help their
blood to clot. These products are obtained by combining components
of blood transfusions from many donors. This placed hemophiliacs
at risk of exposure to the AIDS virus. Now, however, the blood
products are treated to destroy the AIDS virus.

A woman who is infected with the AIDS virus and becomes pregnant can pass the infection on to her child before or during birth.
One-third to one-half of all babies born to AIDS-infected mothers will
be infected and the majority will develop AIDS. Most of these women
were infected through sex with infected partners (bisexual men, hemophiliacs, or intravenous drug users) or through the use of contaminated syringes and needles. Any woman who is planning to become
pregnant and who thinks she may have been exposed to the AIDS
virus should be tested. Women who are infected but do not have
symptoms often go on to develop ARC or AIDS during pregnancy.

A number of health-care workers have contracted the AIDS virus
by exposure to contaminated blood. Some have gone on to develop
AIDS. Health-care workers need to be familiar with safe procedures
and use them routinely.

Most day-to-day behavior does not present any risk of infection
with the AIDS virus. Casual social contact, such as shaking hands,
kissing, hugging, coughing, or sneezing will not transmit the virus.
Sharing towels, sheets, eating utensils, dishes, cups, or straws is not
risky behavior. The AIDS virus cannot be contracted in swimming
pools, hot tubs, or restaurants (even if a restaurant worker has the
AIDS virus and coughs on food). One cannot get AIDS from toilets,
telephones, office equipment, furniture, or door knobs. In most instances it is safe for a child with AIDS to attend school. Each case
should be dealt with on an individual basis, as is done for children
with other serious illnesses. Pets and insects do not transmit the AIDS

virus, and there is no risk in contracting AIDS by donating blood.

If you have any questions or concerns about AIDS, you can get help by calling the Public Health Service AIDS Hotline 1-800-342-AIDS, the National Gay Task Force AIDS Information Hotline 1-800-221-7044, the National Sexually Transmitted Diseases Hotline 1-800-227-8922, or your local health department. Many excellent books are available on AIDS.

Once the AIDS virus has been contracted it is very difficult to predict its course. Some people are able to live for years with the virus dormant in their immune systems. Others get ill within months or years and go on to die. A diagnosis of HIV infection, ARC, or AIDS can be physically, emotionally, and spiritually devastating. People in the prime of their lives are faced with bodily deterioration and death. Sometimes individuals and their families are forced to confront homosexuality and endure the consequences in their jobs, finances, and relationships. Others must deal with an addiction that has become life-threatening. Infection with HIV or the diagnosis of AIDS may result in rejection by an individual's family, friends, co-workers, and church because of misunderstanding, fear, and dogma. A person with AIDS may also feel guilty because of past behaviors that caused the infection.

It is pointless to say that some people are "innocent victims" whereas others "brought it on themselves." All those with AIDS must struggle with the pain, loss, and stigma that accompany this disease. Assigning blame delays healing and serves to separate us into "we" and "they." Healing can occur through acceptance and compassion for those who face this terrible illness.

ENVIRONMENTAL AND OCCUPATIONAL HEALTH

Our focus so far has been on personal behaviors that influence our state of health. The way we choose to live has a great deal to do with our risk of disease and death. But sometimes we are exposed to toxic agents and conditions on the job and at home without our knowledge or consent.

People have always been exposed to hazardous substances in the environment, such as naturally occurring radiation or lead used in cooking utensils. Illness caused by occupational exposures has been recognized for hundreds of years in such trades as mining and chimney sweeping. But during the past 50 years the manufacture and use of hazardous substances has mushroomed.

Americans use more than 62,000 chemicals on a regular basis.[44] Many of them are hazardous. People are exposed to these substances in the manufacturing process, in industry and agriculture, and as consumers. We are all exposed when these substances are disposed of in the environment and they contaminate the air, water, and soil. All of us have small but measurable levels of DDT, PCBs (polychlorinated biphenyls), and certain pesticides in our bodies. No one knows if these levels are high enough to cause long-term health effects.

Unfortunately, a very small proportion of the chemicals that we are exposed to have been tested for their potential effects on humans. Our nation has not spent its resources to examine the possible consequences of the manufacture, use, and disposal of hazardous substances. We are now paying for this lack of concern by widespread contamination and the immense cost of cleaning it up.

Toxic substances cause immediate or late effects, depending on the characteristics of the substance, the dose, the rate of exposure, the length of exposure, and the susceptibility of the individual. For instance, an asthmatic exposed to a high concentration of sulfur dioxide during a smog alert will probably experience symptoms. On a normal day he or she would not feel any effects. A single exposure to a high dose of radon gas will probably not increase the risk of lung cancer, whereas daily exposure to the same dose would be a cause for concern. Someone who is allergic to a substance such as formaldehyde will react to a very low dose, which a nonsensitive person would not even notice.

Environmental pollution is so widespread and involves so many different players that it can be discouraging to begin to examine possible solutions. But we can take actions as individuals to make our homes safer. In the past, lead was used in housepaint and as solder for plumbing. It is possible to have paint and water tested for the presence of lead. Lead is especially toxic to young children and fetuses. It may affect behavior and intellectual development at low doses and cause more severe physical and mental problems at higher doses.[45] Proper lead-abatement procedures are necessary to remove the lead safely. Most local or regional health departments have lead-abatement programs that tell you where to get help. Besides lead, tap water may contain other hazardous chemicals, such as pesticides, that can only be detected by specific tests. State or local health departments can tell you the levels of certain toxic compounds in the drinking water or may be able to perform the tests for you.

There has been much controversy about the potential hazardous effects of radon gas in our homes. The US Environmental Protection

Agency (EPA) suggests that homeowners take action to reduce the level of radon if it is four picocuries per liter of air, or more. Individuals can check the level of radon with a special charcoal canister and then send the canister to a company that reads the radon level. Make sure to use a reputable company. Radon is a known cause of lung cancer in uranium miners and is believed to contribute to lung cancer in smokers and nonsmokers. It is possible to reduce the radon level in the home by improving ventilation in the basement. The EPA has information on where to go for help.

Consumers are exposed to chemicals used around the house, such as insecticides, weed killers, and cleaning products. Although it seems like an inconvenience most of the time, we need to be aware of the proper use, handling, and disposal of these chemicals so we don't cause unnecessary personal and environmental contamination. It may be possible to get along without some toxic chemicals by finding less dangerous substitutes, such as sealing cracks in kitchen walls and using boric acid rather than a strong roach insecticide.

If you live near a landfill where toxic chemicals have been dumped you may want to have your drinking water tested. Your state health department can tell you how this can be done. If you and other people in your neighborhood have illnesses that you think might be associated with the landfill or with another source of pollution, such as an industrial smokestack, you can try to interest the health department in the problem. Most health departments, however, do not have the resources to investigate every geographic cluster of illness. It is possible, however, for you to conduct a simple investigation of your own that might indicate the probability of a real health effect. A book edited by the faculty of the Department of Preventive Medicine and Community Health at the University of Texas called *The Health Detective's Handbook* tells you how to organize your own study of environmental health hazards.[46] If the study is well done and it shows that a health hazard may exist, the health department is more likely to investigate the situation in depth.

As members of communities we need to be concerned about environmental problems that affect us beyond our homes, such as air quality and land use. Many environmental groups can provide information about these issues. We can become involved with these groups in pushing for legislation to protect the environment.

For help with an issue of environmental health, contact your local or state health department, the US Environmental Protection Agency, environmental groups, or schools of public health.

The government requires industry to provide a safe and healthful work environment for its employees and has passed laws and issued regulations to protect workers. Many people have benefited from improved working conditions, but individuals are still being unnecessarily exposed to hazardous substances in the workplace, so we need to be aware of conditions on the job that might pose a hazard to our health.

We can start by looking at our current and past work experiences to determine if we have had any hazardous exposures. "Hazardous exposures" include chemical, physical, and biological agents. A nurse who works in an emergency room may be exposed to tuberculosis, hepatitis and AIDS viruses, and other organisms. Someone in data processing may work in an environment with noisy computers and printers and may come in contact with chemicals necessary for machine maintenance. A woman who works at home will probably use a wide variety of chemicals, some of which may be hazardous, and she may be exposed to naturally occurring radon that seeps into the basement. Occupational exposures include not only chemicals (including familiar ones we use every day) but also noise, radiation, repetitive motion, heat and cold, and bacteria and viruses. Many employees are protected by federal and state worker "right-to-know" laws. Find out if your employer must comply with these laws by contacting your state department of health or environment. For work sites that are covered, these laws require the employer to keep records of all hazardous chemicals and to teach employees about the proper handling of these chemicals. The federal government also has standards for protection from damaging levels of occupational noise and radiation.

Protective measures are often not enforced or our work site does not need to be in compliance, or we may have been exposed before these standards were implemented. To determine whether you are being exposed to a hazardous agent, seek information from your employer, union, or an occupational physician. If you think you were exposed in the past you should inform your doctor so that appropriate testing can be done. Most occupationally related illnesses and conditions, including dermatitis, noise-induced hearing loss, carpal tunnel syndrome, asbestosis, allergies, infertility, cancer, and others, are preventable with the use of currently available technology.

Although it should be the responsibility of government and industry to protect workers, this is not always the case. It is up to us to be aware of potential occupational exposures and to seek out information in order to protect ourselves and others. Help is available from the Federal Occupational Safety and Health Administration

(OSHA), Committees on Occupational Safety and Health (COSH), which are private regional worker education groups, state departments of health, schools of public health, and the Women's Occupational Health Resource Center located in Brooklyn, New York.

Most of us remain healthy in the midst of environmental and occupational exposures. There is no way at this time to determine how much illness is produced by these hazards. We need to be cautious but not overly alarmed about the risks. It is possible to reduce hazardous exposures with current technology. Often these strategies are actually less expensive than what we use now.[47] The question is: How much money and resources are we willing to spend to protect our population from disease resulting from environmental and occupational exposures? We need to weigh this answer against how much we are willing to pay in terms of human health and environmental contamination. We see that cleanup of contamination from nuclear plants will cost $100 billion or more. Toxic landfills that weren't supposed to leak are leaching chemicals into our drinking water and will require millions of dollars to clean up. Many landlords will not spend money on lead abatement and the government does not have the resources or the will to do it. If these issues are important to us we need to let industry and government know. Our risk of illness resulting from exposures in our homes and on the job should be no more than we are willing to tolerate.

SUMMARY

A very diligent medical student went skydiving nearly every weekend. She ate prudently, drank alcohol only occasionally, and always wore her seat belt. Yet, every Saturday or Sunday she drove to the airstrip, strapped on a parachute, and flung herself from an airplane at an altitude of a few thousand feet. Sometimes it seemed she would rather "jump" than eat. After a number of months, she had a particularly bad landing and injured her back. The student was laid up for a couple of weeks, but she resumed jumping as soon as she was able to return her cane to the closet.

We have discussed at length the concept of risk factors and how avoiding certain risks can reduce the likelihood that we will become ill. As we have seen, knowing what is good for us is not the same as doing the right thing. We hear people say that they really enjoy smoking and don't want to give it up, or they'd rather die than have to change their diet, or they forget to wear their seat belts. We have a hard time responding to warnings about health-related behaviors when the consequences of those behaviors are in the distant future. And if we comply with the recommendations we still don't know if it would have made any difference if we hadn't. If I quit smoking at age 30 and die of a heart attack at age 65, did I forgo a pleasurable habit for no reason? Unfortunately, statistics and probabilities apply to groups of people, not to individuals. And it is each of us as individuals who must make daily choices about behaviors that influence our health.

The aim of this book is to help you make informed judgments about the risks you want to take and the consequences you are willing to accept. Taking risks is akin to having stress in one's life. Some stress is good and even necessary to make life worth living. No one can make those decisions for you. This book offers you options that can improve your physical health and well-being. The invitation is for each of us to continue the journey toward wholeness on our own unique path, making choices that maximize good health, deep pleasure, and abundant life.

As we take responsibility for our choices, we realize that as members of families, communities, churches, and corporations, our lives are intertwined. The decisions we make, even the decisions we avoid making, have an impact on other lives. The path to wholeness is never traveled alone.

Part 3

Healing Community

8

Healthy Relationships

People—children, spouses, co-workers, friends, strangers—try our patience, make demands on our time, have opinions and feelings, and sometimes disagree with us. Those we love most of all can be sources of confusion and pain as well as comfort and joy. Life, and particularly "spiritual life," may seem easier without other people around.

The reality is that the discomfort of human relationships draws us into greater wholeness. Perhaps there is divine humor in this. We are stretched by facing life's challenges together. The friction of everyday interaction reveals to us the true nature of who we are. We attract people who reflect us back to ourselves. We "love" or "hate" in others what we do not recognize in ourselves. Or we find ourselves in situations and relationships that call forth from us what we did not know was part of us: strength, perhaps, an undiscovered talent, or perhaps an emotion long denied, such as rage.

Living together in committed relationships forces either growth in consciousness or else determined resistance and life-limiting adaptations. Our children mirror back to us our strengths and our shortcomings, especially those of which we are unaware, either by being just like us or by becoming the exact opposite. Our spouses offer the opportunity of healing our unfinished business with our childhood caretakers or previous spouses by being "just like" others from the past. We may be tempted to bail out, but commitment enables us to move through the difficult times to greater wholeness on the other side.

Relationship problems are actually opportunities to become more conscious and more complete. Personal conflict is a necessary part of our mutual healing. John Sanford wrote:

Through love, anger, and hatred, the powerful, elemental emotions of life, we can be dissolved, injured, renewed and healed, and the process of personality development can take place.[1]

Psychological and spiritual development requires interaction with others. Even those with the specific vocation of consecrated seclusion must be in relationship with the human family. The only way to God is through relationship. The only way to *ourselves* is through relationship.

THE REALITY: ADDICTIVE SYSTEMS

Children are born with a long list of changing needs. Newborns enjoy a primitive spirituality, a sense of being at-one with everyone and everything, based on the inability to distinguish between themselves and others and surroundings. These self-centered newcomers cry to make their needs known. When caretakers respond, babies feel that the world is safe and provident. If their needs are not met, they begin to experience insecurity, frustration, and fear.

Infants gradually make distinctions between self and not-self. They learn whether their smiles and cries are effective, and they gauge the hospitality of the families into which they are born. Children adapt well at an early age to the conditions surrounding them, thus ensuring their survival. The unconscious has an ageless wisdom: even infants recognize truth and penetrate family "secrets." Adaptations to environmental inadequacies can be made at preverbal stages of development, and lie buried in the unconscious, waiting to be triggered by events and experiences of deprivation later in life.

Children have a great many needs and are dependent for a long time. As caretakers we cannot meet all of these changing needs all of the time. We have to be gentle with ourselves as we consider the enormity of the needs of children who depend on us. Also, it helps to have a generous attitude when we consider how our own needs as children were not fully met. The goal is not "perfect" parenting, but "good enough" parenting. With that in mind, we look at the formidable list of needs of children:[2]

Physical care—food, shelter, clothing, touch, protection from physical harm, health care

Nurturing—attention, support, opportunity to realize their potential, love that is as unconditional as we can provide

Guidance—channeling a child's energy and goodwill; role models; learning to serve others; learning moderation and manners; values; learning to be flexible; learning how to relate to their own imperfection with compassion for themselves

Respect—respect for their own and others' feelings; a sense of equality of persons; the experience of being heard and seen and feeling effective; feeling accepted and validated by caretakers; encouragement; sensitive and appropriate affirmation of their gender and sexuality

Education—academic skills; intellectual stimulation; nurturing creativity; vocational training for eventual independent living; development of special talents

Belonging—clear sense of identity as family, ethnic group, faith community; family rituals; bonding in the unique committed relationship as parent and child; stability; invitation to relationship with God

Freedom—open, realistic expectations; empowerment at appropriate ages to take responsibility for self; permission to take risks, make mistakes, and learn

Fun—opportunities to play and to explore; witnessing and sharing parents' love of life; celebration of important events and passages.

The reality is that human caretakers are imperfect. Inadequate parenting by immature parents is common. Severe abuse or incest or parental alcoholism leave gaping emotional wounds, but even those who grew up in safe, loving families have emotional scars from childhood. The most devoted parents in the world cannot meet the endless needs of their children. All children experience deficits.

Healthy systems serve the needs of the individuals within them, and call the individual to full Self-hood and Self-expression. For our discussion, we use the words "addictive" and "dysfunctional" interchangeably to describe social networks that are characterized by the pain of unmet needs, limited emotional expression, or rigidly defined roles. These systems call forth substance abuse, compulsive behaviors, or codependence as efforts to manage the pain.

The words *addiction* and *codependence* have heavy connotations in common usage. The first thing many people think of is alcoholism or drug abuse. Readers are asked to be open to a much broader use of these terms that includes degrees of addiction or codependence, from the subtle to the extreme, and the possibility of being addicted to something other than alcohol or drugs.

Dr. Charles Whitfield estimates that 80 to 95 percent of the population grew up with inadequate parenting.[3] Others in the field of addiction recovery tend toward the higher figure, estimating that over 90 percent of the adult population are addicted and/or codependent, as a result of growing up in dysfunctional (unhealthy) homes. Sharon Wegscheider-Cruse asserts that 96 percent of the population is codependent.[4]

Addiction is "any compulsive, habitual behavior that limits the freedom of human desire," according to psychiatrist and spiritual guide Gerald May.[5] Codependence describes the adaptive behaviors of persons who are currently married or in a love relationship with an addict, persons who have had at least one alcoholic parent or grandparent, *or persons who grew up in homes where emotions were repressed. Substance abuse is* NOT *an essential element of addictive/codependent behavior or dysfunctional families.*

The dysfunctional family is the norm in our culture, and our social systems reflect this sad state of affairs.[6] We simply learn the rules and roles in one dysfunctional setting and carry them with us wherever we go: the workplace, the classroom, the church, government, and international politics. Even those persons who were fortunate enough to grow up in basically healthy families still have to find a way to function within organizations and an entire society that operate as addictive systems.

Our intention is not to blame childhood caretakers for the wounds and adaptations that are part of the human condition. But it is necessary to understand and to name our incompleteness. A compassionate description of the human condition and the need for salvation is found in Gerald May's outstanding book, *Addiction and Grace.* May describes the yearning of the human spirit to love, to be loved, and to move into deeper relationship with the Infinite Source of all love. To love means to suffer. In order to protect ourselves from the pain, we may repress our desire for love, or allow it to become attached to an object. For example, a person may find work more comfortable than risking intimacy with another human being. Addictions, or attachments, capture the energy of our longing for love and restrict our freedom.

The psychological, physiological, and spiritual dynamics set in motion by attachment are the dynamics of addiction. The characteristics of any addiction are increased tolerance, withdrawal symptoms, and self-deception, as well as loss of willpower, and distortions of attention. Addiction of any kind is a form of idolatry that restricts freedom, confuses thinking, erodes self-esteem, and increases the willful determination to have one's own way. May writes: "To be alive is to be addicted, and to be alive and addicted is to stand in need of grace." The question is not whether we are addicted, but to what are we addicted, and to what degree are we addicted?[7]

May observes that addictions are often unconscious; we may notice that we are attached to something only when it causes a conflict, or when we are unable to satisfy the addiction. We can be addicted to anything—a person, a mood, exercise, television, an idea, a food, a feeling, or a value (being helpful, nice, right, famous, rich, and so on). Some addictions attract us to something that is pleasurable or comforting or simply familiar, such as chocolate, approval, religion, hobbies, or worry. Other addictions may be aversive and repel us, such as insects, germs, traffic, public speaking, or certain kinds of people. The problem is that we lose freedom to some degree, and compulsive behavior limits our ability to give and receive love.[8]

A system is a network of persons and processes that are interrelated and function as a whole, such as a family, a group of co-workers, a faith community, a class, a school, an ethnic group, or a nation. The system has an identity and a life of its own, which is distinct from the lives of the persons within it. Each person and interaction has an effect on other members. Systems evoke certain reactions and behaviors from the individuals in the network.[9] (For a review of systems theory and family systems in particular, see chapter 2.)

Addiction is an action; codependence is a reaction; they are two faces of the same coin. In family systems, each person is codependent with the other's addiction. A wife may be codependent to her husband's workaholism; he may be codependent to his wife's need for a distanced relationship. Both have an investment in the status quo; when one begins to change, the other becomes unsettled and anxious. Many substance abuse programs now treat the identified addict and the identified codependent for *both* diseases.

Addictive systems evoke addictive/codependent behaviors. Table 8-1 contrasts the reactions and behaviors called forth by addictive systems and those called forth by healthy systems related to basic core issues: reality, esteem, boundaries, responsibility, power, trust, and freedom.[10]

TABLE 8-1.

Reactions and Behaviors Elicited by Addictive Systems and Healthy Systems

Persons in Addictive Systems	Persons in Healthy Systems
	Core Issues

Reality

Distort, deny, or minimize reality.	Are able to be with reality.
Are cut off from reality, compassion, love by "Don't think, talk, feel" rules.	Are able to feel, to be in touch with heart; able to give and receive love freely.
Feel shame, which impairs ability to form healthy relationships.	Remember that we are human, nothing more and nothing less.

Esteem

Seek esteem from others.	Seek esteem from within.
Feel fear and shame.	Are expansive, full of life.

Boundaries

Experience loss of self.	Cherish others and self.
Become a victim or offender.	Protect self and others.

Responsibility

Feel overresponsible for others' needs; underresponsible for own needs.	Take care of self. Feel worth caring for.

Power

Feel powerless, victimized.	Accept authentic empowerment from within.
Try to control in ways doomed to fail.	Surrender to what we truly cannot control.

Trust

Experience fear, anxiety.	Experience hopeful confidence.
Try to play God.	Let God be God.

Freedom

Attach to objects, persons, processes, or relationships in order to reduce pain.	Are able to detach, love wholeheartedly, and bear the pain of loving and being loved.

Addictions and codependence are often rooted in the suffering of childhood, where basic needs were not met. John Bradshaw writes that codependence is the human response to abuse. Many codependent persons protest, "I was not abused!" However, the opportunities for parents to abandon, shame, or reverse roles with their children are endless: some involve flagrant, shameless disregard for the needs of a child; others are much more subtle.

Healthy parents and caretakers take care of their own needs (for esteem, support, sex, power, nurturance, and the like). They do not use their children to meet these needs. They tend their marriages and do not use children to stabilize them. They allow feelings and expressions of emotion, respect the boundaries of children, and never inflict intentional hurt. Healthy parents and caretakers treat children as unique individuals, not as property. They maintain flexible rules and do not demand absolute obedience. They practice truth-telling and do not lie to children through denial, double messages, secrets, or other crazy-making communication. They do not shame children through abuse, neglect, or desertion, or by using them, invalidating their experience, not caring for their needs, not modeling appropriate behavior, or abandoning them through substance abuse or other addiction such as materialism. Nor do healthy parents and caretakers rob children of their childhoods by expecting them to fill adult roles. Children do not need their parents to be friends, lovers, or servants; they need them to be parents. Conditional love, conditional gifts, or control with money do the same violence to the child's spirit as does control by force or intimidation. Any of these behaviors constitute abuse or emotional abandonment.

Whether the suffering of childhood is profoundly abusive or subtle and infrequent, the child deals with the experience of pain by thinking, "They're okay; I'm not okay." Children depend on adult caretakers for survival and find it intolerable that these responsible adults could do them harm. Inevitably, children take such an experience and translate it into a simple, adaptive, but unhealthy belief, such as: "I'm bad (selfish, stupid, lazy, whatever)," "I'm not good enough," "I should not feel this way," "I have to be good (perfect, right, nice, helpful, whatever)," "I don't deserve anything good," or "Everything bad is my fault."

This belief serves to manage otherwise intolerable feelings. For example, a child has been punished by a teacher for something she did not do and decides that she deserves to be treated this way. Her belief allows her to feel that the punishment is just, and therefore bearable. But her actual experience of injustice, and her feelings, which she has manipulated in order to feel good about the whole thing, do not coincide. The feelings that were consistent with the experience of injustice become "frozen," unfelt, unexpressed, and stored, unconscious, in the body and mind.

When this process happens often in a person's life, and/or the frozen feelings are of significant magnitude, the individual is unable to attain full emotional adulthood. The result is an emotional child in an adult body. Everyone has particular areas in their lives where development was arrested in childhood, somewhere short of full maturity. Usually these areas are very specific and unconscious. Patches of frozen childhood within the psyche cause people to take their unhealed wounds, unfinished business, and subsequent unrealistic hopes into their current relationships. Most people enter relationships as though there is a needy little person inside that keeps hoping that *"now* I will finally get what I need."

Unfinished business can be introduced into a relationship with a friend, a mentor, a boss or co-worker, a pastor, a teacher, anyone, but almost invariably, with a spouse. The unconscious mind seems to seek the perfect person with whom one can heal any unfinished business. Usually this does not happen the way we would like: if only this person would meet this aching need. However, the opportunity for healing is presented when the wound is *repeated*, that is, the other person will *not* take care of the old, unmet need. The person who was so attractive and who once fired hopes for healing will eventually seem like another version of the same old villain. The pain in the present relationship will arouse the feeling that "I've been here before."

A power struggle ensues, as each partner in an intimate relationship tries to get the other to satisfy his or her unmet needs and wishes. In an attempt to get the other to be more loving, each may use self-defeating tactics such as distancing, or angry, critical behavior that only pushes the partner farther away. The cycle can remain unconscious and self-perpetuating for a lifetime, or for the lifetime of the relationship. Relationships often come to an end or the couple may learn to adapt to the situation in ways that diminish the pain, but also diminish life. Very few push through the pain into conscious growth and greater abundance of life. Harville Hendrix offers valuable tools for ending the power struggle and beginning a healthy, conscious relationship in his manual for couples, *Getting the Love You Want*.[11]

One reason why so few relationships realize their healing potential is that the opportunity for healing is not recognized. Two people can look at each other and say truthfully, "This relationship is not good for me or for you. Good-bye." This decision aborts the healing potential of the relationship, when there is no overt physical abuse, mental cruelty, or substance abuse involved. It may be too late, or those involved may be too tired to struggle any longer. However, the awful realization that "this relationship is not good for us" may open the way for honest working together toward wholeness as individuals in order to create a healthier relationship.

The second reason for failed relationships is that the healing process faces double jeopardy. Any relationship or system resists change and tries to maintain stability, and each person inevitably confronts inner resistance to change. Even the person who initiated change will experience anxiety as change begins to take place. Each person in a relationship has an emotional investment, however unconscious, in the way things were. Both individuals need extraordinary courage to break old patterns, become more conscious, feel their feelings, and create a more life-giving relationship.

The choice for healing of addictive relationships places the individual face to face with the unknown. We are so surrounded by dysfunctional systems, one wonders what healthy relationships might look like, and then, how do we get from here to there?

THE VISION: HEALTHY PEOPLE, HEALTHY RELATIONSHIPS

Children who are raised with most of their needs met most of the time by warm, loving, "good enough" parents, have the opportunity to develop into full, healthy adults who can enter into healthy relationships with others.

Pia Mellody describes five major characteristics of healthy adults and how they relate to other persons:[12]

Healthy adults can esteem themselves from within. They feel lovable and trust themselves. There is no need to cling to another person in order to fill their own deficits. Mature adults are free to enter into relationships based on choice and the desire to give and receive love.

Mature adults have boundaries. They know that they are separate individuals. They perceive, believe, and feel separately from others. Disagreement, then, is an opportunity to share different perspectives. They are able to set personal boundaries, to protect themselves from unwanted intrusion from others, and to care for others' boundaries in a nonoffensive, noninvasive way.

Mellody describes adult relationship to reality as the ability to pay attention to one's own body and feelings in order to know one's self. This enables persons to share appropriately the reality of themselves, including their imperfection, with other persons. Those who know themselves are able to have realistic expectations of others, to see one another as human beings, nothing more and nothing less—real people in the real world.

Healthy adults monitor their own basic wants and needs and take responsibility for getting them met. They accept their fundamental aloneness as part of the human condition. This mature approach to dependency and responsibility enables them to choose mutual interdependence with others. Adult relationships are neither overdependent nor antidependent. Taking responsibility for their own needs enables adults to form relationships that do not burden others.

Mellody's fifth characteristic of healthy adulthood has to do with the ability to know and to express one's feelings and needs in an appropriate, creative, effective way. This avoids immature out-of-control chaos, or overmature rigid control. A mature, moderate person is able to be effective and to experience happiness and serenity in a wide range of circumstances.

These characteristics of healthy adult relationships are appropriate with co-workers, colleagues, neighbors, casual acquaintances, members of our faith community, as well as with family and friends. When there is safety and mutual interest, greater intimacy will develop in some relationships. In the deepening intimacy of friendship or romance, there will be mutual self-disclosure, a sense of visibility, excitement, and caring.[13]

When persons are interested in one another, they begin to share their experience of reality with one another. If they meet with a nonjudgmental attitude, empathy, and validation of their feelings (whether the other agrees with them or not), then they feel safe. They become willing to risk more self-revelation and gradually the intimacy between them deepens.

We feel visible when another person listens carefully and responds to us. It is a blessing to be heard and to feel that what we think and feel makes a difference to someone. We are not alone; we have an effect.

Deepening of relationship releases *eros*, or life energy, which may be experienced as excitement, creativity, and/or sexual energy, although erotic energy between persons is not often overtly sexual. Most often *eros* expresses itself in some form of bonding and enhanced creativity.

As relationships become more intimate, the need to express love becomes compelling. Caring for another as for one's self is a joyful form of Self-expression; the heart's desire is to extend oneself for another's growth and happiness. Friends and lovers want to be there for each other in good times and bad. There is much pleasure in time spent together, talking, working side by side, sharing troubles, having fun. Friends devise rituals of friendship; lovers celebrate the sacrament of sex. Love is not sacrificial; it fills us and overflows.

When two mature people freely choose to marry, they make a commitment to one another's growth and development over time. The relationship between two adults who protect and respect and cherish each other forms the ideal crucible for individual growth, for each of the adults in the partnership, and for any children they may have.[14]

In addition to the characteristics of healthy adults and those of intimate relationships that we have described, the adults in a healthy marriage are committed to sharing their whole lives with each other. This involves working at keeping communication clear and open. Both partners should be empathetic toward each other without becoming enmeshed. In a good marriage, partners enjoy sex with each other.

Each partner preferably will have dealt with issues regarding parents and siblings, and previous spouses and children, if any, in order to be able to enter a marriage without old baggage and bindings. Each partner puts loyalty to the spouse above loyalty to the family of origin.

Partners in a healthy marriage are flexible. They are able to give and take, and to adapt or stand firm, and they have the wisdom to know which is called for in a given situation.

A healthy married couple finds a balance between solitude and togetherness. As individuals and as a couple, they reach out to others—children, extended family, and community. They allow themselves to need each other because they love, rather than "loving" each other because they need. And there is the need, in a healthy marriage, for a sense of humor.

*   *   *

Marriage is the cornerstone of a healthy, functional family. What does a functional family look like? A healthy family is the ideal context in which the needs of adults and children can be met. Healthy families are built on the mature, loving relationships of the parents with each other and with themselves.

A healthy family is an open system that offers members the freedom to express themselves as individuals. Permission and encouragement are offered for a wide range of feeling and expression. Communication is characterized by respect and careful listening, and by valuing and trusting each person, using creativity in problem solving, and not having secrets. Each member of a healthy family is invited and supported toward wholeness. The roles and rules in healthy families are flexible, as needs and circumstances dictate.

The family experiences a creative tension between individual autonomy of its members and belonging to the group. A family provides a strong sense of belonging through clear identity, rituals, celebrations, togetherness, play, and teamwork. Yet the family is not isolated; it teaches service to others by reaching out to extended family, community, God, and the world.

Healthy families build self-esteem, value uniqueness, and identify and affirm one another's gifts. They also teach self-discipline, self-care, and self-love. All in all, the healthy family provides for the physical, emotional, social, intellectual, and spiritual needs of the individual and of the family as a whole.

Some health-promoting guidelines for the family include these concepts:

Everyone is good enough.

Everyone is a gift.

Everyone is lovable and capable.

Everyone has a right to develop to potential physically, emotionally, spiritually, and intellectually.

Everyone has a right to experience feelings and to express emotions in a nondestructive way.

It is okay to talk about problems.

Children may disagree with adults.

No one is to be hurt deliberately.

Mistakes are opportunities for learning and growth.

* * *

The vision of healthy persons in healthy relationships offers a goal to move *toward* rather than simply having a negative experience to move *away from*. However, we soon realize that awareness and desire for change are not enough. As we come up against resistance to change from an addictive system or from within ourselves, we find that willpower alone is not the answer. We are divided. We want freedom, but something strong and deep within us still needs our addictions and codependence to relieve our suffering. Simply deciding to change will not produce change that lasts. What will?

THE CHALLENGE: HEALING OF RELATIONSHIPS

The cycle of addictive/codependent behavior is self-perpetuating. The way out of the endless cycle is to do the unexpected thing:

If we want to take charge of our lives, we need to acknowledge our dependence on God. We tend to get our power issues backwards; trying to control what we cannot control, feeling helpless where we are actually empowered to become responsible. When our attempts to manage our pain and to control our situation fail, we come to the place of freedom. Exhausted by our own efforts, humbled by failure, too weary to continue with our old patterns, we have "no choice." Although this place feels like "no choice," we always have a choice; to continue with our compulsive behaviors, to intensify our own efforts, or to turn to God for help. What feels like defeat is the hidden passage to new life. It is when we cry out "I cannot change myself; I need salvation," that the change we seek has already begun. God's help waits for an opening into our lives. When we "give up," we give God room to heal us. We are not our own saviors; God saves.

If we are out of touch with our emotions, we can work with the body. The body offers physical cues that tell us what is happening in us emotionally. Physical activity that focuses awareness on the body can be very helpful. For some, noncontact physical activity such as t'ai chi ch'uan, yoga, dance, running, walking, swimming, or tennis are helpful. Others benefit from contact therapies such as massage, acupressure, acupuncture, or therapeutic manipulation.

A way to get in touch with our bodies is to recover the child in us. Children are naturally unself-conscious and at home in their bodies. We can look at childhood pictures, and recall childhood pleasures, friends, games, songs, and trips. If we feel much sadness about our childhood, we probably still have wounds that need healing. A popular T-shirt reads, "It's never too late to have a happy childhood." As adults, we can now reparent the wounded child within us.

If we learn to take care of ourselves, others will care for us in ways that are healthy and respectful, not rescuing or overly responsible. When we value ourselves and others, we attract persons who value themselves and others. Those who value themselves inspire confidence: that is, there is no need to rescue or be overly responsible for those who can be trusted to take care of themselves.

To become the best we can be requires that we make mistakes, because when we make mistakes, we learn that we are trustworthy. When we err, misstep, or do something "wrong," we experience a healthy self-correcting part of ourselves that does not want to repeat the mistake.

If we are in conflict with someone we love, we can dare to "lose." It is by *not* "winning" that everyone wins. Win/lose situations indicate a power struggle in which each person competes to be the victim of the other's wrongdoing. We can look at our own contribution to the problem. We can learn to listen to one another carefully. We can get help if the problem is too emotionally loaded to handle alone. Chances are that we are trying to tell each other the truth and neither of us wants to hear it.

If we are tired of an addictive behavior that has become self-defeating, we can practice it consciously. We can learn to appreciate what this behavior is trying to do for us, observe all of our feelings about it, and forgive ourselves for needing it. A behavior that is performed consciously will produce self-correcting feelings. The addictive behavior may be overeating, procrastinating, lying, gambling, smoking, seeking perfection, avoiding intimacy, watching television, or even abusing a substance. Whatever the behavior, we avoid our deeper feelings about it as long as we try to apply willpower to resist it. The pattern of resistance and failure creates feelings of frustration, shame, and guilt. Resistance and temporary success evoke feelings of pride and the illusion that "I can handle it." On the other hand, doing the behavior consciously allows deeper feelings to surface. We soon realize that this is *not* what we want. We also come face to face with our need for salvation; we cannot conquer even the smallest addiction by ourselves.

Then we can be understanding about the need for the addiction and compassionate toward ourselves for being addicted. In inner dialogue, our conscious, adult selves might say to our addictions: "Thank you for protecting me and preserving me until I could deal with the reality of my life. You have served your purpose. Now I need to face life without dulled feelings and senses. I want to be more whole, more alive. I want God to be God in my life. With God's help, I will now take over the task of caring for my wounded self." As we care for ourselves by getting help, by reparenting ourselves, and through healing prayer, the addictions, no longer needed, will gradually fall away.

Rather than dulling reality with addictions, or adapting to painful situations with codependence, the challenge is to be with reality.

The way to clear present relationships of unfinished business from the past is to let the reality of the past into our awareness. Instinctive coping mechanisms such as denial, distortion, or minimizing, once served to protect us from pain that we could not handle. Eventually, when these coping mechanisms create complications greater than the suffering they relieve, it is time to give them up. When the truth of the past is allowed to enter into awareness, when we can identify legitimate needs that were not met, we are enabled to experience authentic feeling about those unmet needs. These feelings of frozen anger and grief can be released.

The thought of confronting the past and its feelings can be frightening and explains why many hesitate. However, thawing frozen feelings releases their energy for change and healing. It empowers us to care for ourselves and for others. Feelings are the means by which we perceive reality: to the extent that we are cut off from our ability to feel, we are prevented from perceiving reality as it is.

Anger is problematic in our culture. We tend to be afraid of anger for many reasons. We are taught that anger is the opposite of love, and that anger is often associated with violence. We are afraid that we are unloving and unlovable when we are angry. Anger at caretakers was intolerable when we were children and the fear of anger continues into adulthood.

Anger is protective of ourselves and of our loved ones. It alerts us that something is happening that is injuring us somehow. Anger can be a "red flag" that tells us to pay attention to what is going on, to name the situation as accurately as we can, and to choose an appropriate action to correct the situation. Far from being the opposite of love, anger is a self-loving, justice-loving, self-caring response. It becomes a problem when it is ignored, and bottled-up inside, and then finally erupts in a destructive, overreactive episode because it has not been dealt with in a healthy fashion all along.

Frozen anger leads to despair and alienation. It is necessary to feel old anger and to express it appropriately in order to experience empowerment and forgiveness. It is moving *through* our anger that we can come out the other side; it is by using the energy of anger, that we can go beyond victimization to self-care.

Frozen grief is numbing. The pain of unmet needs, the losses through death, divorce, or the whole range of emotional abandonment, remain lodged in the psyche and soma, interfering with our ability to feel and to be fully alive. Experiencing our grief enables us to feel more fully in the present, so that we can perceive the present reality more accurately.

If frozen emotions are frightening to us, we do not have to face them alone, nor do we have to face them all at once. A good therapist and/or support group can facilitate the healing process and offer reassurance along the way.

It is important as well to allow the reality of the present to enter our awareness in order for us to make free and responsible choices and to have healthy relationships. The persons with whom we are in relationship today are not going to satisfy unmet childhood needs, nor will they respond favorably to childish tactics. We have to give up unrealistic expectations and connect with the anger, sadness, and/ or grief we may experience about the present also. Only then can we open to the other persons in our lives and be able to receive them as they are, rather than as we want them to be.

Help is available through individual or group psychotherapy, 12-step programs, self-help and support groups, and marriage or family counseling.

Through individual or group psychotherapy with a qualified, competent therapist, we can learn to deal with unresolved issues from the past, thaw out frozen feelings, and learn how to be with and to channel feelings that were once too overwhelming to bear.

Twelve-step programs are based on the foundational principles of AA (Alcoholics Anonymous). They include Al-Anon for spouses and family members of substance abusers, NA (Narcotics Anonymous), OA (Overeaters Anonymous), and GA (Gamblers Anonymous).

Many groups are forming across the country for ACOAs (Adult Children of Alcoholics) and ACODF's (Adult Children of Dysfunctional Families). These include therapy groups, self-help groups, and 12-step self-help groups. Many ACOA groups also welcome adult children of dysfunctional families in which the dysfunctions of the family of origin include nonalcohol as well as alcohol-related dynamics. Many people may turn away from valuable help, not recognizing themselves as addicted and/or codependent because they and their loved ones do not use alcohol or drugs. Every family that is affected by alcoholism is dysfunctional, but alcoholism is not the central issue in every dysfunctional family. A wealth of insight and support is available to adult survivors of dysfunctional families through ACOA and ACODF programs, educational books, and other 12-step programs.

Marriage or family counseling that looks at the family as a system, and deals with unresolved issues from the family of origin of the adults, offers the best opportunity for long-term healing. We can ask any potential counselors about their approach and trust our instincts in finding one that is right for us.

Our relationships with others and with God depend upon the health of our relationship with Self. We must tend to unhealed wounds from childhood, otherwise they become powerful determining factors in our present relationships. The frozen feelings of unhealed wounds limit and distort our perceptions of present reality. The myth of a happy childhood, or a miserable one, shields us from the whole story, and from our integrated wholeness. In order to recover our true Selves, it is necessary that we remember.

Either/or, all-or-none thinking protects us from letting in the reality of childhood experience. If we have any tendency to think "My childhood was okay" and to dismiss any memories of pain as inconsequential, or if we think "My childhood was awful" and overlook memories of warmth and nurturance as irrelevant, then we protect ourselves from the whole truth. For most people, the truth is that childhood was mixed: good times and bad, shame and encouragement, nurturance and rejection. Letting the whole story into our awareness enables us to sink deeply into our own human experience and to be in touch with the child who felt all of these feelings, the child each of us once was.

Why would we want to know the joy and suffering of the child once again? The inner child is the repository of the originally blessed person we were created to be. The child is unself-consciously at home in the body, able to sense and to feel with uncanny accuracy. The child who feels safe is spontaneous, playful, expansive, and affectionate. The child who feels unsafe becomes cautious and self-protective. The child instinctively takes care of self and expresses love generously. The inner child also blesses us with a sense of wonder.

One often has to pay a price in suffering in order to enjoy the fruits of a healed inner child. At St. Luke Health Center, many health-care participants found that getting in touch with the child within included getting in touch with the pain of having received inadequate parenting. The good news is that, as adults, we can love the wounded child within ourselves and heal any inadequate caretaking by engaging in play and prayer, and by taking care of ourselves.

Playing with dolls or stuffed animals, reading children's books, listening to music, playing games, or going to a circus or the zoo sometimes enables persons to get in touch with the child in them. Trusted friends may be willing playmates, or this healing play may be shared with a child who is part of your life. Some people choose a doll or toy to represent the inner child and take care of the doll as they want to care for the child within, holding it, loving it, rocking it. We can talk to the frightened or angry or wounded child within us, through speaking, praying, or writing a journal. When we feel the inner child's feelings, whether they include anger, fear, helplessness, sadness, or whatever, the adult part of ourselves can speak reassuringly to the inner child. The child needs to know that the adult will care for and protect him or her.

The healing stories from our faith traditions give us a way to understand our experience and to pray through it. For a Christian, healing stories from the Gospel, such as Jesus raising the centurion's daughter or the widow's son from the dead, can be vehicles of praying for healing of the child asleep or "dead" within us. Or the parables of Jesus, such as the story of the Good Samaritan, who cared for the man beaten and abandoned half-dead by the side of the road, can offer a way to pray for the frozen child abandoned and left for dead earlier in life.

By becoming tender caretakers of ourselves, we invite the wounded inner child to come out, grow up, and thrive. Those persons who have been taught to put everyone else's needs first must work hard to learn how to identify their own needs and get them met. Self-care honors the preciousness of the person God created us to be. Far from being self*ish*, caring for oneself creates opportunities for others in the social networks around us to be more mature, responsible, healthy, and whole as well.

Finishing work on family of origin or other early issues frees us of the legacy of the past and enables us to live into the present. We can form grown-up, empowered, truthful relationships with those in our lives: parents, siblings, spouses, children, friends, extended and blended families. Recent books that explain the dynamics of unfinished business and offer tools to reclaim our lives include:

Codependent No More, by Melody Beattie

Toxic Parents, by Dr. Susan Forward, with Craig Buck

Recovery: A Guide for Adult Children of Alcoholics, by Herbert L. Gravitz and Julie D. Bowden

Getting the Love You Want, by Harville Hendrix, PhD (for couples)

The Dance of Anger and *The Dance of Intimacy*, by Harriet Goldhor Lerner, PhD (especially for women, but helpful to men, too)

Facing Codependence, by Pia Mellody, with Andrea Wells Miller and J. Keith Miller

Healing the Child Within, by Charles L. Whitfield, MD[15]

The effort put into self-care, the courage required to walk through our old pain, and the suffering entailed in facing once unbearable reality are richly rewarded in abundant life, new freedom, new depth of feeling, and particularly, a deep feeling of trust in one's self, God, and life in general. The journey toward wholeness is worth the cost. *We* are worth it.

SICKNESS, HEALTH, AND CHANGE IN THE FAMILY

The presence of physical illness tells us nothing about the spiritual journey of the person who is ill, or about that person's family and other social networks. Sickness happens in healthy systems and it happens in addictive systems. Sickness occurs in persons who are working toward wholeness and in persons who are relatively unconscious of the inner life. Many people are relieved of physical or emotional suffering as they become more conscious, empowered, responsible, and self-caring. Physical or emotional disturbance occasionally seems to get worse before it gets better as the body releases forgotten memories and frozen feelings. We cannot make assumptions about ourselves or anyone else because an illness develops.

The new-age concept that each person creates his own reality has too many people suffering "new-age guilt" when they get sick. Would-be helpers may inquire about the lessons one needed to learn from this experience, or suggest that a particular chakra may be blocked, or diagnose a sick friend based on illness as a metaphor. (Ear problems? What is it that you don't want to hear?) Although there may be some truth to each of these approaches, a problem develops when we follow the human tendency to generalize: if it's

true once, it must be true all the time. This is not so. These generalizations based on partial truths send a potent, counterproductive
message: if you are sick, or stay sick, there must be something spiritually wrong with you. This kind of thinking is hardly an advance
over the notion of illness as God's punishment. Some new-age think-
ers make gods of people and blame them for their own disease. This
is not compassion.

Each of us is incomplete and in need of healing. Illness does not
constitute an invitation to diagnose or judge our neighbor. We may
see someone's "blind spot" where growth is needed for improved
health, but perhaps that person's denial or unconsciousness is firmly
in place. These defense mechanisms are valid self-protection, needed
for reasons we do not know. To attempt to dictate the timing of
another person's growth or to define it is an act of arrogance. We
would do well to remember the teaching of Jesus: that it is hypocritical
to observe the flaws in others while overlooking our own shortcomings.[16] We may not see our own "blind spots," but rest assured, we
have them.

It is true, however, that illness frequently occurs under certain
circumstances. Knowing that, we can make choices which enhance
disease prevention, or if illness occurs, we can look for clues which
enhance healing. When people see the factors involved in their own
illness, they are free to assess their resources, their readiness to
change, and then make a conscious choice: to move toward wholeness
or to wait; to prepare for growth or to withdraw into self-protection.
It is okay to be wherever one is now. God loves each person unconditionally.

At St. Luke Health Center, the staff frequently observed illness in
persons who occupy "malignant positions" in a family system; people
going through periods of change, loss, or transition in their lives;
persons with a backlog of repressed feelings; or those observing anniversaries of losses or holidays that trigger memories or feelings.

"Malignant positions" are those roles within the family with the
greatest vulnerability to illness.[17] (See chapter 2, especially "Social
Dimension: Illness within the Family System," for a review of family
systems theory and malignant positions.)

In a healthy family, individual members are able to think, feel, and
act separately from one another. Since family members do not over-
react to one another, the healthy family system is better able to tolerate
stress. In dysfunctional families, family members are constantly
checking one another's "emotional temperature" and reacting ac-
cordingly. Stressors create more disruption for dysfunctional families,

which in turn causes more frantic reaction in an attempt to manage the stress and restore some sense of equilibrium. We can think of healthy families and dysfunctional families as opposite ends of a continuum: most families are somewhere on the continuum, partially healthy, partially dysfunctional.

All family systems unconsciously seek to manage stress and to restore equilibrium when the stability of the system is threatened. In families in which members are less able to become separate, or self-differentiated, stress in the family system increases vulnerability to illness. For example, illness in one family member may take the focus of attention away from another stressful situation or relationship. A family member may become ill in an unconscious attempt to get other family members to "change back," or stop defining themselves as individuals. Or a newly differentiating family member may become sick rather than risk becoming a new self, with all of its costs and rewards. For healing to take place, family members can be helped to become less reactive to one another and more able to function as separate individuals within the family system. Also, attention must be brought back to the source of chronic anxiety within the family.

Change, loss, or transition of any kind challenges a family's ability to adapt, whether the change is subjectively positive or negative. Even a small change is a crisis to a family that is dysfunctional. The more disruptive the crisis, the greater is the possibility that an illness may develop within the family in order to manage the stress. It is easier for a family to integrate stress in one part of the system than in the system as a whole. Chronic illness, alcoholism, eating disorders, underachieving, overachieving, perfectionism, moralism, procrastination, grandiosity—any disease can locate the chronic anxiety of the system in one family member. For healing to take place for the individual and the family, receptive family members need to be coached and supported in behaviors that are not reactive to the emotions or to the illness of other family members. This breaks the pattern of reactivity to one another, and draws the focus back to the source of chronic anxiety.

Emotional repression is a common characteristic in persons with life-threatening illnesses. Dr. Lawrence LeShan found that 76 percent of cancer patients in his study, as opposed to 10 percent of the control group without cancer, tend to cover up their despair and not to communicate their anger, hurt, or hostility to others. They typically experienced stressful childhoods, characterized by poor parent-child relationship, which leads to low self-esteem and hopelessness. Their sense of self-esteem comes from outside themselves and they depend on others for validation, approval, and love. Many of these people manage their feelings so that they will be liked—and they are. "He's the nicest person!" is commonly heard in response to the news that someone is ill. Or, "she is the sweetest, happiest person I know." People whose emotions are repressed are more vulnerable to illness following the loss of an emotional mainstay—a spouse, a significant other, a meaningful job, a home. For healing to take place, a person may need to be encouraged to be less "nice" (i.e., less people-pleasing) and to be more expressive of emotions, even the ones that may make others uncomfortable. The emotions that are resisted are usually the more aggressive, self-assertive, self-caring ones. Health requires taking care of self rather than taking care of others' feelings; people are responsible for their own feelings.[18]

Anniversaries and holidays sometimes trigger old feelings or unresolved issues that lie buried in the unconscious. A pattern might evolve: at a certain time each year "something" happens—an illness or injury or depression or job loss. The person can investigate what happened that time of year earlier in his or her life in order to find a clue to what calls for healing. Perhaps a loss occurred, such as the death of a parent, or a divorce. An illness or other crisis may occur when an individual reaches the age when a parent died, or when one of his or her children reaches the age at which the individual experienced a trauma in his or her own childhood. The unconscious remembers and seeks healing of forgotten wounds.

Disease can function in one's life in a number of ways, ranging from coping mechanism, to catalyst for change, to disaster. Serious illness is a major crisis that can totally disrupt the life one has known and causes the person to face every part of life anew. As one reintegrates his or her life to include the illness, the experience of change may be positive or negative or mixed. Illness is not to be romanticized as a glorious opportunity for personal healing and growth; for some it is, for others it is not.

Serious disease in any family member has a profound impact on the family. Life-threatening disease causes people to face their own mortality and to reevaluate their priorities. In many cases, people decide that their family is very important to them. The illness experience may include not only the disease itself but also such hardships as pain, suffering, loss of employment, debts, worry, changes in self-image and body-image, changes in roles, and shifts in power within the family. Some families are drawn together and made stronger by the experience; other families are destroyed. There is nothing romantic about a family crisis of this proportion.

When someone we love is faced with serious illness, it seems not to matter whether the cause is genes, or pollution, or stress, or childhood wounds, or an inability to care for one's self, or anything else. What matters is loving one another and being with one another in ways that promote life and promote healing.

We can develop implications for health promotion, based on our knowledge about family systems and some of the conditions of particular vulnerability to illness. The guidelines are the same whether the goal is disease prevention or well-being in the presence of sickness in the family:

1. We need to live our own lives. When one person in a family system retains or improves individuality and well-being, the whole family benefits.
2. We need to be proactive rather than reactive. We must define ourselves—thoughtfully choosing our own actions, based on our own values, feelings, and needs, rather than reacting to the approval or disapproval of others—and take responsibility for those choices.
3. We need to communicate feelings in a way that is respectful and that invites others' response. Healthy people are in touch with reality and with their feelings. They speak for themselves.
4. We need to set priorities and to live as though life is precious. We all have limited time; mortality is a fact of life.
5. We need to take care of ourselves. Even when a family member is sick, we must first be responsible for meeting our own needs. This principle is based on trust that our needs *include* the need to care for loved ones, but that is not our only legitimate need in times of crisis, or any other time.
6. We need to give and receive help. People generally want to help one another, particularly in a crisis. We can be specific about what we need when friends ask what they can do for us; we can be specific about what we can offer to others in need.
7. We need to be childlike. Healthy children are unself-conscious, spontaneous, loving, playful, free, accepting, and full of wonder. They are themselves.
8. We need to stay connected with others. We must be able to give and receive freely, and to share the joys and burdens of life with one another. It is *being with* one another that is mutually healing.

Arthur Kleinman describes the social experience of chronically ill persons and their families as a movement "back and forth through rituals of separation, transition, and reincorporation"[19] as the diseased person moves in and out of family involvement, in and out of health-care facilities, and in and out of normal everyday life. There is always uncertainty—about one's health, one's sense of power, one's constantly changing relationships.

When illness does occur, a positive outcome can be enhanced by remaining connected with one another within the family, and making the effort to keep the family connected with the larger community. Illness tends to be a self-absorbing experience for the person who is sick. Chronic and/or serious illness often isolates the patient within the family and isolates the family within the community.

A person who is sick needs to be included in the life of the family as much as possible. Sharing events of the day, including a sick person in discussions and group decisions, and keeping isolation to a minimum enable the person to participate in family life. This reduces the demoralizing feeling of simply being a burden. People need to be needed.

Families affected by serious illness or injuries have to make a special effort to stay connected with support systems outside of the family. Social networks may include close friends, extended family, church groups and clubs, neighbors, and casual social contacts. People cannot offer support or practical help if they do not know there is a problem. And once they do know there is a need, they have to be told what specific help is needed. Perhaps a neighbor can help with transportation and errands; a close friend can listen to feelings; extended family can help with child care; other friends can help with meals; everyone can support the family with prayers and encouraging words. It does require an effort to consider the relationship, what is needed, what may feel intrusive and what feels genuinely helpful, but it is worth reaching out to others. Most people want to help.

Staying in touch with God and self can be difficult in a health crisis that affects ourselves or our loved ones. Sometimes we need to rely on the faith of others around us to carry us through a particularly difficult time. Many stories of healings in the ministry of Jesus describe how the faith of family and friends made healing possible. We do not have to believe for ourselves all the time. When, for example, a loved one lies desperately ill in a hospital bed surrounded with monitors and IV's and tubes, we might pray with all our hearts, or we might be unable to imagine God's existence or benevolence at all. We can only cry out from the truth of what we are feeling now—if that is fury, or doubt, or pleading, so be it. God can take it.

The key element to becoming a healing community for one another is vulnerability. Jean Vanier, Henri Nouwen, and other assistants to handicapped persons in L'Arche communities have eloquently described their discovery that God is revealed through the weakest, the poorest, the powerless, and the most broken of persons. Families and communities are gathered around the most defenseless ones who evoke our most tender care. The infants and children, elderly, handicapped, and infirm people are the ones who provide the reason for our commitment. They are the ones who provide the push we need to work for reconciliation and unity; it is their love and their need that often hold the community together. As they awaken what is tender and reverent and loving in us, we are mutually healed.[20]

Community is a two-way street. Vulnerable people put us in touch with our own vulnerability. The innocent, pure, trusting love of a little child reaches through our self-protective barriers and calls forth the wellsprings of love. We become more accessible, human, peaceful, and nonviolent. Our hearts of stone become hearts of flesh. God is revealed both in the vulnerability of need and in the vulnerability of compassionate response.

Sometimes we can *do* nothing about the suffering of another except to *be* in solidarity with them. The challenge is to be open enough to let in whatever experience is at hand, with its light and its darkness, its joy and its anguish, in order to receive its blessing. Like Jacob, who wrestled with God until the break of day, we will be changed, though we may walk away with a limp.[21]

9

Healing Presence

SELF-LOVE

"Love your neighbor as yourself." This central teaching of Jesus may be restated, *You can only love your neighbor as much as you love yourself*. If you want to love others more, you must first learn to love more of yourself.

Any "love" we give while we dislike aspects of ourselves is not love at all, but an attempt to fill our own emptiness and to feel better about ourselves. How different it is to serve others out of the desire to give from one's true Self. This love does not require anything in return: no need to congratulate one's self or to indebt the receiver. Distinctions between giver and receiver disappear; neither one is superior to the other. Both persons give and receive simultaneously. The giver offers help and receives the gift of having the offering accepted. The receiver accepts what is needed and gives welcome to the love that has been extended. Each must be generous to the other in order for creative, liberating love to occur.

Our ability to love others depends on growth in self-love, which includes becoming aware of and learning to love what is hidden and unattractive in us—the wounded, ugly, impoverished, murderous, and foolish. By acknowledging these parts of ourselves, we cease hating them in ourselves or in other people. Otherwise, we risk becoming alienated from others whom we judge negatively, because we are alienated from the same things in ourselves.

It is important to love what is good in ourselves as well: our better qualities, talents, appearance, whatever we like about ourselves. We are likely to deny our positive traits as well as our negative ones.

Knowing ourselves as we really are diminishes our tendency to protect a false image. There is no need to pretend to others or to ourselves that we are more or less than human ("hero or zero," as one friend puts it). Dropping pretenses frees us to attend to the needs of others because we know that we are needy, too. Thus we are free to love our shared humanity.

Holiness is not perfection; it is wholeness. *To be healthy and to be holy is to be human.* The fully human person contains a whole cast of characters, some of them loving, some wounded, some violent, some creative. As fully human persons, we recognize that we are creatures of God, interdependent with each other, and that we are guests at the generous banquet of life.

If we want to participate in the banquet and to care for our fellow guests, we must first care for ourselves. Sometimes that means saying "no" to a legitimate request in order to care for our own need for solitude, rest, family time, friends, or prayer. Caring for our own needs increases our capacity and desire to be available to others, with less risk of burning out. We become more expansive and generous when we take care of ourselves.

Self-love creates an environment of mutual safety, respect, and care. For example, if those who seek our help know that we avoid over-extending ourselves, they need not fear that they are imposing. They can receive what help we can offer as a free gift, with no hidden strings, costs, or obligations. The encounter can be a mutual blessing—two human persons meeting in love, both giving, both receiving, both being healed.

COMPASSION

When we come to know ourselves as we truly are, we know that nothing human is alien from us. The longing for love, the fear, the loneliness of our neighbor is our own longing, fear, and loneliness. The pain of the oppressed as well as the tyranny of the oppressor can be found in our own hearts. We discover that we are capable of anything. If I know my own alienation, loneliness, hope, fear, sadness, love, and hatred, and accept them, I can look with compassion on others who are just like me.

Compassion involves openness: the inner hospitality to receive another person into our hearts; the willingness to feel another's pain and to extend ourselves in personal concern; and the willingness to be changed by our encounter with another.

Compassion means creating an open, nurturing, creative space for another person. There is a close relationship between the Hebrew words for "compassion," *rachum* or *racham*, and for "womb," *racham* or *rechem*. Compassion means offering a womblike space, setting self-interest aside to make room for the other to reveal herself or himself and to grow. Inner housekeeping creates space for another, by cleaning up preoccupations, hurts, jealousies, and angry feelings. Then we can give full attention to the one we receive as guest.

Clearing space within is only the beginning of true inner hospitality; our guests need safety for healing and growth to take place. Safety depends on a nonjudgmental attitude, a sense of equality, and empathetic presence. No sane person is going to risk self-revelation to someone who may judge him or her negatively. Even a positive judgment can be hurtful because it still implies that the "helper" enjoys a superior position that permits judgment. Healing encounters take place between persons who know they are equal, though one may be in a helping role at the moment.

The word *compassion* is derived from the Latin words, *com-*, "together," and *pati*, "to suffer."[1] We suffer together when we open our hearts to the pain and the wonder of one another's experience. "Being with" one another is healing. We cannot truly *be with* one another without an emotional response. A teddy bear or an affectionate pet offers more comfort and healing than does an emotionally distant person. Anyone who wants to help must risk experiencing pain—the other's pain, and his or her own. Henri Nouwen describes a positive, life-giving martyrdom, which involves giving one's life for another in his book, *The Wounded Healer:*

> Real martyrdom means a witness that starts with the willingness to cry with those who cry, laugh with those who laugh, and to make one's own painful and joyful experiences available as sources of clarification and understanding.
>
> Who can save a child from a burning house without taking the risk of being hurt by the flames? Who can listen to a story of loneliness and despair without taking the risk of experiencing similar pains in his own heart and even losing his precious peace of mind? In short: "Who can take away suffering without entering it?"[2]

There is a popular notion that a helper's feelings must be left out of a helping relationship. On the contrary, we know that personal concern is very healing. We can bring ourselves into a relationship and acknowledge the sadness, hope, helplessness, concern, anger, and caring that we feel within ourselves in response to those who share their experience and pain with us. This establishes a living connection that can be a crucible of change and healing for both.

A relationship that is healing for the one who seeks help will also produce change and healing in the one who offers helping presence. We risk being changed by the encounter. If the helper is unwilling to be touched by the relationship, it will not be healing for either person.

Connecting with one another and with the suffering of humanity gives meaning to personal suffering. Stephen Levine teaches that if we let go of identifying with "my pain" and enter into "the pain," we can break out of the isolation that pain can create. Helpers can facilitate letting go of unnecessary suffering and enable deepening the unavoidable suffering to the level where it is shared with all humankind. We discover that we are not alone in our pain, but that all persons are together in "the pain" of our shared body and shared heart within the Great Heart of God.[3] Henri Nouwen says in *The Wounded Healer:*

> When we are not afraid to enter into our own center and to concentrate on the stirrings of our own soul, we come to know that being alive means being loved. This experience tells us that we can only love because we are born out of love, that we can only give because our life is a gift, and that we can only make others free because we are set free by [God] whose heart is greater than ours.[4]

Self-love requires Self-giving. And those who give themselves to others in compassion find that their inner hospitality, personal concern, and emotional responsiveness can find active expression through communication, healing touch, visualization, and healing prayer.

COMMUNICATION

Communication creates human bonds. Sharing our stories with one another and listening reverently to others' experiences are forms of love. Speaking in a way that shares one's self requires a willingness to risk vulnerability; listening involves opening our eyes, ears, and hearts to receive one another.

We have a deep human longing to be heard and understood. Unfortunately, genuine sharing and listening are rare. When warm, interested, caring listening takes place, both speaker and listener are blessed.

Healthy, life-promoting speech is honest. Offhanded social lies such as "how are you?"—"fine," when one may not be feeling fine at all, create discord within one's self and block communication. Healthy communication is based on congruence, the state in which body, mind, spirit, thought, speech, and action are in agreement.

This does not mean that we should express everything we think or feel. Judgment needs to be exercised in how, when, and with whom we will share our struggles, hopes, and consolations.

When we express our thoughts, feelings, ideas, and experiences, we give our lives and ourselves to one another. This is not a simple matter of ventilating, or letting off steam, but an act of generosity and vulnerability. Self-revelation occurs when we stop pretending, when we allow our inadequacies and strengths to show. There is an immediacy in healthy communication. Old feelings are not bottled up until they erupt, but are processed thoughtfully as they occur. We simply tell our own story in our own voice.

Storytelling heals. As we tell the narrative of our personal experience, we claim the experience and allow it to change us. We become more ourselves in the process. The healing potential of storytelling can be increased by connecting our personal story with larger stories, such as the sacred stories of our respective faith traditions, or the universal stories found in mythology, folklore, and great literature. The larger stories provide road maps for our journey, showing us the way, the pitfalls, and the meaning.

Both speaker and listener share responsibility for effective communication. The speaker risks self-revelation; the listener invites, makes an effort to understand, explores, clarifies, and seeks to identify the hidden needs of the speaker.

Listening is a highly disciplined form of love. One must put preconceptions and preoccupations aside in order to receive what the other is saying. Listening attends to the other's needs. Morton Kelsey writes: "When we try to love without first knowing the needs of those around us, we are likely to be ministering to our own needs and not to theirs."[5] However, when we do listen to another's needs, we are able to receive the gift that person is.

Communication in any significant depth requires a climate of safety and mutual respect that involves both inner and outer aspects. A safe inner space is free from the threat of judgment, free from preconceptions, free from hidden agendas, free from one-up, one-down distortions in relationship. A nonjudgmental, open, balanced, mutual encounter allows healing to take place. The outer physical space is important, too. Privacy, freedom from interruptions, sufficient time allotted, and comforting surroundings put people at ease. Confidentiality is essential. A person's story is a sacred trust and it is to be protected and treated reverently.

Listening is *not* problem solving; it is *not* removing the pain; it is *not* taking on others' burdens; nor is it an opportunity to feel better about one's self. Problem solving promotes distancing. One person becomes the expert and the other becomes the inept. It is usually not possible to take away another's pain and generally not what the person is asking for. Listening does not change the situation—the struggle, or grief, or pain will most likely continue—but understanding and entering into another's experience make the difficulty less lonely and somewhat easier to bear. Taking on others' burdens is a symptom of the disease of overresponsibility—helpful to no one. Listening in order to feel superior, helpful, comparatively fortunate, powerful, or all-knowing is a perversion of healing listening. It may soothe one or both parties temporarily, but it will not last, and soon another "fix" is needed.

Listening that helps and heals involves being a companion, not a teacher, guru, parent, or rescuer. Simply being present, entering into another's experience, understanding, and caring may feel like "doing nothing," but it is exactly what others want most. We may want to *do more*, but it is *being with* which heals.

Helpful listening is not "doing nothing," it is *work*. The effort of attention is a form of service. It requires putting self aside in order to focus mental concentration, care, and consideration on the other. All kinds of thoughts, related ideas, similar experiences, distractions, or self-centered responses try to capture our concentration. We can gently observe them and allow them to float by in our consciousness, neither fighting them nor being captured by them. When we notice the presence of distracting thoughts, we can simply call our attention back to the one to whom we listen.

We associate listening with ears and hearing, but other senses are valuable sources of information, also. We listen more thoroughly if we utilize our eyes and our hearts as well as our ears. Words are just one mode of expression. Those who tell their experiences may use nonverbal, visual modes of communication in addition to words. Smiles, sighs, gestures, appearance, posture, degree of relaxation, openness, eye contact, presence or absence of enthusiasm, strength— all of these and other nonverbal cues either support or conflict with verbal messages. When verbal and nonverbal messages contradict each other, a good listener can feed back that there is a mixed message and ask for more information.

Listening with one's heart requires attention to what is happening within the listener as well as attending to the other person. The listener's feelings, including any physical reactions, are automatic and truth telling. They are reliable sources of valuable information about ourselves, the other, the situation presented, and the relationship.

Genuine care for another includes making ourselves available through honest feedback. We all know how much it means to receive a heartfelt word of encouragement, affirmation, or sympathy. Even anger, sadness, or disagreement can be amazingly valuable coming from someone who cares. Each of us longs for personal reaction from those who are willing simply to be human and to be in touch simultaneously with their own hearts and ours.

Participative listening is an act of love, that is, it involves extending one's self for another's healing and growth.[6] Listening leads to other forms of love in a ripple effect. Listening is a gateway to empathy, that ability to enter one another's experience, to see with his or her eyes, and to feel with his or her skin. Empathy creates a desire to give active support, which means lending our emotional or physical energy to another's needs, including expressing the other's concerns to God through prayer and communicating God's loving presence back to them.

A word on conflict resolution—sometimes there is disagreement. When we limit our conversation to naming our own experience, our needs and feelings, argument is unlikely. Often when someone tries to make someone else see things the same way, creating a right/ wrong, win/lose situation, an argument develops. One person blames another and the situation degenerates into a contest of who is the victim of the other's wrongdoing or wrong-thinking. Perhaps another person or a community might enter the situation in an attitude of peace to facilitate conflict resolution. Each person in conflict needs to open willingly to the experience of truth. If that is not difficult enough, each has to take equal responsibility for whatever is happening in the relationship. Both have an investment. When both claim responsibility (ability to respond) and are willing to experience the truth, even if it is painful, the conflict evaporates and a new challenge takes its place. Then there is a right/right, win/win situation with a solution in which both can receive some of what they want.

Good communication leads to deepening intimacy. At first our risk taking in self-revelation is measured carefully. We talk about safe subjects first, perhaps an idea, a book, a movie, cars, or sports. If this feels safe enough, we may speak about things that mean more to us and begin talking about feelings. If we are received with reverent listening, our trust grows, and our fear of hurt, abandonment, or disappointment diminishes. As we relax into another's acceptance, we may take greater risks, sharing our darkness, our deepest wounds and fears. Within relationships characterized by caring, acceptance, and a nonjudgmental attitude, both speaker and listener often find themselves resonating in sympathy, much like living heart cells placed in contact with each other begin to pulsate in unison.

Sharing the struggle and pain in an individual's life can be a dark passageway into the light of the Holy. At the center of each person, beneath the layers of personal experience, illusion, and pain, we find the Holy of Holies, the sacred place wherein we meet God. Only those who stay present to all levels of self-revelation, courageously facing the other's pain, and feeling the pain of caring, can enter the sanctuary of another's soul. The "wounded person" suddenly seems translucent, radiant, pure, and ageless—angelic! Perhaps this is what "eternal life" looks like. As privileged witnesses, we stand in awe; the one whom we have "helped" has become a God-bearer to us.

TOUCH

Our skin relates sensitively to people and environment. Skin responds with pleasure or displeasure to the weather, textures, touches, food or chemicals we have ingested, sexual excitement, stress, pollutants, and benevolent or hostile energies around us.

Many of us are starving for caring touch, yet cultural taboos inhibit the natural flow of human physical contact. Touching persons of the same sex arouses fears of homosexuality. Touching persons of the opposite sex may be misinterpreted as a sexual come-on. Touching strangers, touching yourself, touching elderly or handicapped persons, touching someone in authority, touching an employee, touching family members, touching to sell, touching to communicate power— all have elaborate codes of prohibition. These unspoken rules constrain our freedom to offer healing touch to those for whom we care.

It helps to remember that we all need to be touched with love. It is well known that babies fail to thrive, and sometimes die, when they do not receive enough stroking, cuddling, holding, or loving. We forget that the same is true of elderly persons who may appear too fragile to touch (or who may stir up our fears about the fragility of our own lives). Teenagers are often deprived of touch because their developing sexuality arouses fears in the adults who care for them. Noticing one's own appreciation of a teenager's youthful sexuality, without resisting those feelings of appreciation, enables parents to hug their children, or to give a pat on the back, without fear of becoming inappropriately sexual. One might speculate on how much teenage sexual activity and resulting teenage pregnancy are the result of touch deprivation. Handicapped and sick persons find their opportunities for giving and receiving life-giving touch diminished by isolation and by physical barriers, such as bedrails, walkers, and wheelchairs.

Adults often seek physical affection through sexual intimacy. Although this is an excellent way to experience loving touch, it is not the only way. Hugging, holding, dancing, stroking, massaging, and cuddling are options, depending on circumstances and relationship. We need touch, even during periods of voluntary or involuntary celibacy. It is a mistake to avoid physical contact simply because sexual expression may be inappropriate, undesirable, or unavailable.

Our hands can communicate the love that we feel for another person. In verbal communication it is important to be in touch with our own feelings and to give clear messages; the same is true of the powerful nonverbal communication of touch. It is important to be sensitive to the wishes and boundaries of the person to whom we want to communicate our care by asking what physical contact is wanted and needed and what feels good.

A person's receptivity to physical contact depends on familiarity, timing, pain, and relationship dynamics. A presumption that it is permissible to touch a particular person may be met with a bristling reaction if the contact is perceived as patronizing, overly familiar, infantilizing, or falsely comforting (i.e., denying feelings). Respect for the individual is critical. If permission to touch is not already established in a relationship, it is best to ask if touch is agreeable to the other person, either verbally ("May I hold your hand while we talk?") or nonverbally (extending an open hand for the other to respond).

Most of us who are not in physical or emotional pain welcome physical affection. Touch is comforting; it relaxes and connects. It expresses emotional support. Often we are able to face the challenges of life more readily when we receive physical and emotional support.

Persons who are ill need to feel needed, too. Persons who are elderly, sick, or handicapped need to feel included in life. One of the beautiful things about hugs and other kinds of physical affection is that we give and receive at the same time. Everyone has an opportunity to give; everyone receives; everyone experiences a little bit of healing.

Touch is life-giving. We see this depicted in Michelangelo's inspired ceiling of the Sistine Chapel. He shows God imparting life to Adam with a fingertip to fingertip touch. Similarly, we experience a continuation of the same mystery whenever we lovingly touch one another.

Some highly developed cultures base their healing systems on the movement of energy through the body. In a healthy person, the energy flow is balanced and smooth. Thinning of the energy field around the body, blockages, or dissipation, which are disruptions in the flow of energy, make a person more vulnerable to illness. Restoring balance to the flow of energy enhances healing of sickness that may have developed as a result of the disruption. The meridians through which energy flows and energy centers, known as chakras, were mapped out thousands of years ago.

Controlled experiments indicate that something beneficial occurs when energy-based healing methods, such as acupuncture, acupressure, and Therapeutic Touch, are employed. Western science is at a loss to explain how this works. Some suggest that it is a placebo effect, or that peripheral nerves may be stimulated which in turn cause the central nervous system to release endorphins, which are natural painkillers. Alternatively something may occur electromagnetically, although the fields are so subtle that their effect defies explanation. However, we know that these techniques *do* work. Touch-healing reduces anxiety and tension, reduces pain, and very often speeds the healing process.[7]

At St. Luke Health Ministries, we did not wait for technology and scientific method to catch up with the wisdom of the East and of African and other so-called primitive cultures. We have used ancient and modern, secular and religious energy-based methods as well as Western medicine with beneficial results. Acupuncture, massage, laying-on of hands, hugs, and hand-holding have been an integral part of our program of treatment and prevention of disease for those participants who are open to touch-healing.

Within relationships that are characterized by mutual respect and trust, physical contact seems to promote a healthy exchange of energy. For example, welcome hugs seem to balance energy and give huggers a "lift" (and hugs are readily available without a prescription). We are responsible for getting our own needs met. Don't wait for a hug to come to you; go out and give and receive what you need.

Giving or receiving physical caring reminds us that each of us is a body-self. Connection with our own physical reality enables us to be in touch with the physical reality of others. To be in touch with the physical reality of other persons, animals, plants, and the planet herself increases our capacity to care deeply. An expanding spiral of compassionate, embodied care-giving is set in motion. Societies that are open to physical pleasure and who enjoy the body, and raise their children with a great deal of physical nurturance, are peaceful, cooperative societies. Conversely, societies that suppress physical pleasure and raise their children with little physical nurturance produce violent adults.[8] One way to peace is through giving and receiving nurturing, pleasurable physical contact.

VISUALIZATION

Imagination is powerful medicine. Words, thoughts, and beliefs create expectations and images that affect our health. Depending upon our expectations, the body's natural defenses may be mobilized to enhance healing, or they may be suppressed, which could jeopardize the healing process. Expectations that increase fear result in a stress reaction which suppresses the immune system. Expectations that increase hope marshal the self-healing abilities of the body and call the immune system into action.

For example, if a person with a life-threatening illness believes that the situation is hopeless, then the course of the illness is likely to follow this expectation. It is possible to die of the diagnosis, rather than of the disease, when terror or despondency result from a grim prognosis. If, on the other hand, a person with the same serious illness is given reason to hope and feels empowered to respond, or continues to hope despite what has been said, the body's ability to heal itself is greatly enhanced, and "miracles" sometimes occur. The expectations we hold are critically important to our health.[9]

The imagery of visualization can affect the immune system, which is very responsive to imagination. Endorphins and enkephalins are natural chemicals produced by the body that produce powerful medicinal effects, particularly in blocking pain and boosting immunity. These two categories of "feel-good" chemicals are associated with happiness, humor, and hope, and are often experienced in connection with music, laughter, running and aerobic exercise, with eating sweets, and helping others. Imagery which increases happiness, humor, and/or hope produces the same physical effect.

Relaxation and imagery, the two elements of visualization, can be used to promote health and boost the healing process. Relaxation reduces the "fight-or-flight" response to the threat posed by illness.

When stress is reduced, the energy and resources of the body become available for healing. Imagery refers to mental representations that are preverbal, that is, without language, and which invoke the senses, especially sight. Visual imagery refers to the mental pictures that run through our minds like a movie. The imagery employed in visualization involves deliberately creating positive mental images of desired results.

Akhter Ahsen theorizes that all experiences are stored in memory as eidetics—vivid, lifelike, mental images, which remain constant, so they can be retrieved from memory. An eidetic has three components: (1) an image, or mental picture; (2) a somatic state, or physical and emotional feelings; and (3) a meaning, or cognitive interpretation of the event.[10] According to David Cheek, emotional traumas and severe stress become encoded in the mind in a form of spontaneous hypnosis.[11] This learning is typically forgotten (becomes unconscious) and can be accessed and changed only through an altered state of consciousness.[12]

The altered state of consciousness that naturally accompanies deep relaxation allows access to encoded memories and learning. When we become conscious of the beliefs that inform our bodies, we can evaluate the images associated with our beliefs and change them to more life-promoting images if needed. The mind can reframe any problem in a way that moves toward resolution and healing.[13]

Relaxation and altered states of awareness affect blood chemistry dramatically. Relaxation exercises produce changes that are the exact opposite of those produced by the "fight-or-flight" response. Whereas prolonged stress tends to depress the immune system, relaxation tends to enhance it. At the very least, a healthy state of balance, homeostasis, is restored, and the relaxed person is better able to set the imagination free. The relaxation and imagery of visualization form a complete cycle. Relaxation frees the imagination that then has access to the body through the altered state produced by relaxation.

Early pioneers in exploring the mind-body connection, including Franz Alexander, Walter Cannon, Hans Selye, and Milton Erickson, have made significant contributions to understanding how attitudes, beliefs, perceptions, emotions, and experiences are processed by the body and translated into biochemical and physiological change. Researchers have demonstrated that images and emotions affect physical reactions, and physical reactions reciprocally affect images and emotions. Each thought, memory, and emotion is a biochemical and electrochemical activity within the brain and nervous system of the body.

Thus thoughts, memories, and emotions affect every cell of the body.

The nervous system is divided into the somatic nervous system and the autonomic nervous system. The somatic nervous system (SNS), often called the "voluntary nervous system," is the part of the nervous system that enables us to interact with the outside world through verbal language and musculoskeletal movements.

The autonomic nervous system (ANS) regulates such internal functions as waking and sleeping, eating, body rhythms, temperature, respiration, heartbeat, blood pressure, blood chemistry, glandular activity, and the immune system. Although the ANS has been referred to as the "involuntary nervous system," a signficant body of research confirms that the mind has much more control over these physical functions than was previously believed. The ANS is divided into two overlapping systems, the sympathetic branch, which prepares the body for action through the "fight-or-flight" response, and the parasympathetic branch, which maintains normal, internal stability and balance between organ systems.

Imagery is preverbal. It affects the body with or without verbal, cognitive interpretation by the left hemisphere of the brain. Researcher Jeanne Achterberg hypothesizes that nonverbal imagery is the only language that the ANS understands and that all mind-body communication with the ANS must be translated into images.[14]

The part of the brain associated with the storage of images (the right hemisphere in most persons) and the part of the brain associated with emotional response (the anterior frontal lobes) are richly connected to the limbic-hypothalamic region of the brain. The limbic system is the processing center of emotions. It is also connected and interactive with the hypothalamus and the ANS. The hypothalamus is the regulatory center of the internal environment, and along with the pituitary gland, the "master gland" of the body, with which it is in constant chemical dialogue, the hypothalamus regulates the entire ANS. Therefore, many researchers conclude, as does Ernest Rossi:

> The "limbic-hypothalamic system" of the brain is the most obvious anatomical candidate for the role of connecting mind and body. Indeed, it is a unique psychophysiological communication channel between the expectations and creative processes of mind and the emotional physiology of the body.[15]

For further reading in this exciting arena of mind-body healing, we suggest *Imagery in Healing*, by Jeanne Achterberg, *The Healer Within*, by Steven Locke, MD, and Douglas Colligan, and *The Psychobiology of Mind-Body Healing,* by Ernest Lawrence Rossi.[16] Also outstanding and readable are the books by Herbert Benson, Joan Borysenko, Barbara Brown, Norman Cousins, Jerome Frank, Michael Harner, Kenneth Pelletier, and O. Carl Simonton, Stephanie Matthews-Simonton, and James Creighton.

Imagery can address the symptoms—the headache, cancer, ulcer, rash, and so on—or it can address the encoded learning, if we are conscious of it. Imagery that addresses encoded learning can be life changing. Instead of imaging a disease and the body's defenses, one could visualize healing an emotional wound. Those who felt abandoned or neglected as children and who seek to have those needs met could visualize the inner child being rocked and cradled and stroked and receiving the care that is needed. As adults, we can each parent our own inner child through the gift of imagination. Those who feel helpless could visualize themselves as capable and strong, able to develop solutions to problems, and able to care for themselves. Those who feel worthless could affirm their own dignity as human beings and visualize themselves believing that truth.

Whether a physical cure takes place or not, some healing is always possible. It is a significant accomplishment to heal such old, life-limiting beliefs as: "I don't deserve anything good," "Nobody loves me," "Everyone abandons me," "I'm worthless," or "I'm helpless," "The world is unsafe," "Everyone is against me," or "I'm not good enough." Sometimes changing these unconscious beliefs leads to a physical cure, sometimes it leads to deep, abiding peace. Either way, it is "miraculous."

Embodied beliefs, images, and valuable unconscious material can become conscious in a variety of ways. Recording your dreams and keeping a journal are helpful (chapter 3). Bernie Siegel and others use artwork to understand the inner world of the individual in treatment.[17] The individual is then empowered to make responsive choices.

Complete instructions for visualization can be found in *Getting Well Again,* by O. Carl Simonton, MD, Stephanie Matthews-Simonton, and James L. Creighton.[18] The element of prayer may be added as a matter of personal faith and preference.

Those of us who have faith in a religious tradition have additional resources at our disposal. We can combine the tools for healing, self-love, compassion, communication, touch, and visualization, with the elements of faith and openness to the grace of God. This is the experience of healing prayer, for ourselves, for others, and for our world.

HEALING PRAYER

Healing prayer is a courageous act of love for ourselves and for others. It is daring to say "yes" to life and "yes" to truth, no matter what the cost.

Too often praying is a form of wishful thinking. For example, someone who smokes heavily prays to be spared from lung cancer. We cannot ignore our bodies and then pray to survive our own neglect. That is praying to be rescued from the consequences of our actions. If we are tempted to pray for things to change magically and painlessly, we are praying for relief, not for healing.

Praying for healing does not mean giving up and doing nothing. The popular exhortation, "let go and let God," may seem like an invitation to abdicate our ability to respond to life. Instead, it admonishes us to find a balance between two paradoxical truths: (1) that we are in need and dependent upon God, and (2) that "God helps those who help themselves." We have to work on those aspects of our lives over which we do have control and trust God to sustain us through circumstances beyond our control.

Healing prayer is a risky business. It requires self-knowledge, being in touch with our heart's desire, opening to the Holy, and willingness to be changed by that encounter.

Self-knowledge involves experiencing our own humanity, including our vulnerability and need, as well as our dignity and worth. True humility enables us to stand in right relationship with God and with one another, and to face the reality of the present situation. We are connected to one another in our vulnerability and incompleteness. If we feel complete and in charge, we have no need of God or one another; if we experience debilitating shame, we are cut off from God and one another by a sense of worthlessness. Self-knowledge enables us to open to a power greater than ourselves and to reach out to one another as fellow-travelers on the path to wholeness.

Being in touch with our heart's desire enables us to be unambiguous in presenting our need to God. Sometimes we can be in pain and not really know what we want. It requires considerable effort to figure out what the pain is about and to identify exactly what we need. When we are in touch with the specific need, we feel our yearning physically and emotionally. We can then articulate the need in prayer.

Visualizing the desired outcome is a powerful adjunct to verbal prayer. We cannot have what we cannot imagine; we have to set the imagination free to create images of the abundance that Scriptures tell us is God's will for us.

Jesus challenged his disciples: "Everything you ask and pray for, believe that you have it already, and it will be yours."[19] To create an image of a desired outcome and then to believe that one has already received it may feel like an exercise in self-deception. But holding the image of desired outcome in mind is an exercise in self-direction. The process of creating an image requires us to identify specifically what it is that we want. We present our heart's desire in images and words of prayer, and God within and around us responds.

We may have the need and the imagination, but feel intimidated by the question of "how much faith" is required. The Scriptural answer is amazing: only the size of a mustard seed![20] God simply needs a small opening into our lives.

Opening to the Holy means giving God room to work. God respects our boundaries, barriers, and free will. When we pray for healing, we enter into intentional relationship with God and with God's people. Authentic relationship involves a *willingness to be changed* by our interaction with the other. Our willingness to be changed by our encounter with God opens the way for God's will to be done. And God's will is wholeness.

We can create space for the Holy in a number of ways, for example, prayer, meditation, dreams, journaling, the arts, and ritual. (Review chapter 3, especially "Encountering the Spiritual Realm" and "Classical Spiritual Disciplines.")

Daring to trust creates the opening for change—and healing—to occur. Gerald May writes that it is faith that enables us take the risk of opening ourselves to God in times of vulnerability, weakness, and pain:

> It is where our personal power seems most defeated that we are given the most profound opportunities to act in true faith. The purest faith is enacted when all we can choose is to relax our hands or clench them, to turn wordlessly toward or away from God. This tiny option, the faith Jesus measured as the size of a mustard seed, is where grace and the human spirit embrace in absolute perfection and explode in world-changing power.[21]

We exercise this "tiny option" when we pray for healing. (Paradoxically, the "tiny option" is often experienced as a "leap of faith.")

When we risk turning toward God, we create space for the Holy One, who desires our wholeness. But we do not control the Other, and we may be surprised by God's Spirit, or be "broad-sided by grace," as one friend expresses the experience. This little space within us characterized by our willingness, the size of a mustard seed, becomes the meeting ground of the human and the Holy.

Divine life fills us from within and around us, changing our lives with illumination and power. The light of God's presence often brings insight, which may take the form of an intuition, a verbal message, or an image. The insight may cross over into consciousness from the unconscious of the one seeking healing, or through anyone in the healing community praying for that individual. God's in-filling grace also brings energy for change. The new light and energy may be experienced as subtle or astounding or anything in between. God knows what we need at the moment. As we are increasingly enlightened and empowered, we begin to experience change of mind, change of heart, and change in our bodies.

As we integrate new insights and images, our self-image changes, as do our perceptions of our circumstances and relationships. We naturally begin to experience different emotions than we did before our encounter with the Holy. The body is very responsive to images, thoughts, emotions, and perceptions; somatic changes begin to occur. Healing always takes place when we pray: both healing and prayer diminish unconsciousness and promote wholeness. As healing takes place, the body responds. This can lead to improvement or even a cure of physical disease.

Whether physical cure takes place or not, a chain reaction of healing is set up by one individual's encounter with the Holy. As one's self-perception is altered, emotions and behaviors change. This has an impact on relationships and social networks. Addictive systems are disrupted and challenged by the presence of a healthier member. Others will have to make choices, to resist or to grow.

Healing prayer may take the form of prayer for our own healing, corporate prayer for healing, or intercessory prayer.

Personal Prayer for Healing. The fact that we pray for healing is transforming in itself. We dare to place our needs before God in hopeful expectation, and we present ourselves as receptive to change. We can pray simply in our own words, or we may use the repetition of a word, phrase, or short prayer from our faith tradition with our breathing. One variation of personal prayer involves combining such a word or phrase with the Relaxation Response, a technique that

Herbert Benson, MD, calls the "Faith Factor." Research affirms the powerful effect of personal religious or philosophical beliefs, and suggests that we "may well be capable of achieving remarkable feats of mind and body that many only speculate about."[22]

Each faith tradition has its sacred writings through which people experience the truth and grace and power of God. Just as Christians call Jesus the Word of God made flesh, we find that the word of God continues to be made flesh in each of us through prayer. By repetition, the word or words of our prayer take root in our hearts and in our lives, healing us, transforming us beyond anything we could have asked or imagined.

Corporate Prayer for Healing. When a community prays for one another's healing, the power of prayer is multiplied. The people present offer themselves, their time and their love, for the healing of one another. The loving connections between persons enrich the prayer experience. Spoken prayers evoke insights and images, which frequently spark the healing potential within the individuals. The concern of a loving community envelops the person seeking healing, lending support in time of need. Those who pray for others are also touched and healed by the energy that flows through them. The experience of everyone participating is frequently one of extravagant love: our love for one another, plus God's all-embracing love, flowing in abundance far greater than we have the capacity to receive.

All of the elements of healing that we have identified in chapter 3 and this chapter are readily incorporated into communal prayer for healing. These include the recognition of need, consecrated place, prayers of confession, focused attention, self-love, compassion, communication, touch, visualization, and an openness to change as well as placing ourselves and our needs before God. The senses become engaged through laying-on of hands and anointing with consecrated oil. Listening to Scripture, silent reflection, prayer, singing, and meaningful symbols enhance openness to the sacred. Communal prayer is a whole-person experience.

Intercessory Prayer. We can also pray effectively for loved ones in their absence. Time, distance, and even death pose no barriers to the power of prayer. When we pray for another person, the relationship expands to welcome God's healing love into the relationship, in addition to our own.

Intercessors are those who pray on others' behalf. This kind of prayer involves being in touch with someone's need and bringing that need before God. We may find that we naturally carry our loved ones' needs in our heart and prayer. Sometimes, we feel called to pray for a person or a situation that simply comes to mind when we are quiet. Intercessory prayer is a commitment; therefore, we must be attentive to the leading of God's Spirit in order to discern for which of myriad needs we are called to pray.

We need not be concerned about *how* to pray for ourselves and one another; prayer for healing is simply a matter of carrying one's own or another's needs in our hearts and opening our hearts to God. Whatever we need, whatever we feel, whatever our faith, or doubts, or fears, or hopes—this is our prayer. Our own words will do just fine.

Anyone can pray for healing. The fact that healing is a special gift or vocation in the lives of some persons should not scare others away from healing prayer, any more than the special talent of a fine singer or exceptional cook should be a reason for others to avoid singing or cooking. Healing is a gift that God wants to give. God *needs* us to participate in order for healing to take place. We have to let go of our insecurities, pride, false humility, and other barriers so that we can offer ourselves as instruments of God's healing. Each of us can be a connecting link between the physical and nonphysical realms, offering our bodies, minds, hearts, our whole selves as a vehicle for the Infinite Holy One, who is the source of all life.

"Worthiness" is not required for effective healing prayer; in fact, God can do some of the best work with "broken tools." Often people will say, "I want to be healed so that I can be a channel of healing for others." Certainly some healing is helpful—just enough to know from experience that God is the healer, to recognize healing when it occurs, and to be with those who seek healing in compassion and equality. Complete healing is not a prerequisite, thank goodness, or no one would be qualified. Mindfulness of being incomplete and on the way toward wholeness is an asset. We remember that God is God and that we are God's creatures. "We are only the earthenware jars that hold this treasure, to make it clear that such an overwhelming power comes from God and not from us."[23]

The healing process usually takes time, whether one prays for physical healing, an emotional or spiritual healing, the healing of memories, or the healing of a relationship. Healing may occur faster than we imagined possible, or slower than we hoped for. God's timetable may be different from ours. We must persist in prayer, trusting that God's will is healing, and that healing is, in fact, taking place.

We need not protect God from "failure" by never asking for anything. *Prayer always heals.* To pray is to change; at the very least, the one who prays is changed. We cannot offer ourselves as channels of God's healing power without being touched and healed by that power in the process. Those for whom we pray are touched, supported, and healed by our prayers. When we pray for ourselves, we deepen our relationship with the true Self within us. In all cases, God defines the healing. We can expect something wonderful, even if the healing we receive is different from the healing we requested.

According to a Hasidic tale, a man was suffering greatly, so he went to his rebbe for words of comfort and healing. "I am desperate," the man said. "My world is falling apart. I don't know what to do. The pain is unbearable. Please help me—you are my only hope."

And the rebbe responded with compassion: "I cannot help you out of the thicket, because I am caught up within it, too. But I offer you my hand and if you will come with me, at least I can lead you more deeply into the thicket."

God waits for us in the depths—of ourselves, one another, our experiences. The journey toward wholeness is a shared venture. Not only are we all in this together, but God is with us. Our dreams, meditations, relationships, beloved places, art, music, play, wonder— all beckon us to enter our experience more deeply. The emotions that stir us, causing us to smile through tears of sorrow, or to weep with joy, invite us to know that there is more. We can share with each other what we have learned along the way about health, healing, and wholeness, but in the moment of truth, there is only the truth of the moment. We are not alone.

Conclusion

T he six facets of the wholeness paradigm have a profound impact on how we think about health promotion and disease prevention:

An *integrated, nondualistic approach* to personhood demands whole-person health care. Interdisciplinary teams can address diseases of body, mind, and spirit in an integrated way, and also recognize the individual's illness experience.

Keeping God at the center requires a reordering of values, so that medicine, expediency, or economics do not become ends in themselves.

A *systems approach* encourages a macroscopic view of the factors involved in any person's health or sickness. Disease, then, is viewed as a symptom; treatment addresses causes in addition to the medical aspects, increasing the likelihood of a lasting cure.

The *interfaith* dimension allows persons of all faiths, or no faith, to apply the wholeness paradigm to their lives, honoring their relationship with God, and their feelings within and about that relationship. Everyone has faith in something; part of the healing process involves finding out what that is, and facilitating the personal search for meaning in one's own experience.

This paradigm extends *inclusivity* by avoiding sexism, and also by remembering that all persons are equal and valuable, regardless of their gender, age, ability, race, sexual orientation, economics, or education. This invites us to stretch our thinking, and to seek definitions of mental, spiritual, and physical health which allow for differences. The young, able-bodied, middle-class, white, American male cannot be the standard of physical, mental, and spiritual health for all persons.

An *ecological, creation-centered approach* calls us to responsible interaction with a highly interactive and sensitive ecosystem. From the ecosystem of the single cell in the human body to the ecosystem of

233

the planet, nature has a limited ability to tolerate abuse and a limited ability to recover. We must care for the natural world.

As we apply the wholeness paradigm to issues of health promotion and disease prevention as we have throughout this book, we begin to see staggering implications. What we need is a revolution, beginning with how we think, but moving beyond to how we live and interact as members of families and faith communities, as providers and users of a medical system, and as citizens of a powerful nation and a global community.

The family would become a place where whole and separate selves can thrive and grow and care for one another. This sometimes occurs through the friction of daily living, which can be a crucible for growth, but it always occurs through mutual respect, nurturance, affirmation, and empowerment.

Faith communities would invite and support growth, rather than sheltering those who would seek to avoid it. They would offer stories that heal, and witness to God's healing presence, as sources of meaning and remembrance of God's faithfulness.

Our health-care system must change to one that truly cares for wholeness. Superspecialized health care has failed us; too many people do not have access to adequate care, and those that do have access often find themselves caught in a system that is bewildering and unresponsive to their needs. To reduce fragmentation, we need whole-person health-care teams staffed by primary care practitioners who can address diseases of body, mind, and spirit in an integrated way, and who take the individual's illness experience into account. The inequitable distribution of care is a national disgrace; every person has a right to whole-person care, regardless of his or her financial resources.

Our present medical system is disease-oriented, expensive, inequitable, and sometimes adversarial. Human and financial resources are overwhelmingly devoted to finding cures for disease, rather than advancing preventive medicine and public health; *both* are important. We spend an enormous amount of money on medical care and yet millions of people are without health insurance, and infant mortality rates among some minority populations rival those of developing countries. The fear of malpractice suits fosters an adversarial climate that results in higher fees, fewer services, and many unnecessary tests.

Health care should be prevention-oriented. In terms of human suffering, and often cost-effectiveness, it is better to prevent disease than to cure it. Research and training in prevention must be funded. Collaboration with health educators can have a tremendous positive impact on public health. The cost in loss of life, the inability to work, the cost of treatment, and the suffering for preventable diseases and injuries is inestimable. As a society, we can provide incentives for prevention by, for instance, pressing for insurance coverage for prevention services, encouraging insurance premium discounts for nonsmokers, facilitating work site health promotion programs for all workers, and insisting on meaningful labels on processed foods.

Health-care practitioners have an obligation to provide humane treatment with the consent, understanding, and input of the individual treated. The patient must be included as an involved member of the health-care team. At the same time, the issue of responsibility must be dealt with in a sensitive, nonblaming manner; the health care consumer is able to respond and to be involved in his or her own treatment.

Similarly, as citizens, we are not to blame for the state our health-care system is in, but we are responsible for helping to change it. As members of a political body, we need to provide equal access for all persons, not only to health care but also to education, employment, housing, and basic human dignity. There is an urgent need to end the genocide in our cities, reservations, and economically depressed areas that is caused by spirit-killing unemployment and poverty, inadequate education, substance abuse, homicide, lack of health education, and inadequate health care. Looking to heal the wounds within our own national borders is not enough; we are accountable for our actions and exploitation in other countries as well. The United States is just one member of a global family.

The earth is our common home. We must protect the fragile ecosystem and concern ourselves with peace in our world. Peace begins within each person. It is easier to see how the world needs change than it is to understand that by changing ourselves, we change the world. Each of us must choose life through integrity and faithfulness in the small things, from moment to moment, day to day. As we pursue our own healing in this manner, we contribute our individual little grains of wholeness to those of other fellow travelers, until we will all see and share a new creation.

Notes

PART 1. BODY, MIND, AND SPIRIT

CHAPTER 1: CHOOSE LIFE!

1. We learn that we are not unconditionally lovable, nor is it safe to love unconditionally, from collective beliefs. In general, there is a collective agreement that we are all separate; that some persons, traits, and experiences are more valuable than others; that some people have more rights; that time is our master; and a host of other illusions. The cost of these socially accepted agreements is that we are forced to adapt. This adaptation involves agreeing to the illusions, living in fear, needing to control, being unable to trust, experiencing conflict, and wanting. These are core issues for every human being in this finite world.

2. John A. Sanford, *Healing and Wholeness* (New York: Paulist Press, 1977), p. 19.

3. Bernie S. Siegel, MD, Lecture at Omega Institute, Rhinebeck, NY, Aug. 29, 1987.

4. Carl G. Jung, quoted in Sanford, *Healing and Wholeness*, p. 105.

5. Bernie S. Siegel, MD, *Love, Medicine and Miracles* (New York: Harper & Row, l986), p. 4.

6. Ibid., p. 66.

7. Zeph. 3:17–18.

8. Ps. 139:17–18.

9. Bernie Siegel, Omega Institute, 8/29/87.

10. *The New Brown-Driver-Briggs-Gesenius Hebrew and English Lexicon* (Lafayette, IN: Associated Publishers and Authors, 1978).

11. Ibid.

12. Ibid.

13. The human dimensions described by modern psychology as the drive to self-actualization, the transpersonal, and collective unconscious, including archetypes, would be included in the non-physical aspect of personhood, which the authors of this book call spirit.

14. *Brown-Driver-Briggs-Gesenius Hebrew and English Lexicon.*

15. Arthur Kleinman, MD, *The Illness Narratives* (New York: Basic Books, 1988), concept pp. 3–4, quote p.6.

16. World Health Organization, quoted in: Kenneth L. Bakken, *The Call to Wholeness* (New York: Crossroad, 1986), p. 8.

17. Benedict Ashley and Kevin O'Rourke, *Health Care Ethics* (St. Louis: The Catholic Health Association of the United States, 1978), p. 33.

18. Stuart J. Kingma of the Christian Medical Commission, quoted in Bakken, *The Call to Wholeness*, p. 8.

19. Ashley and O'Rourke, *Health Care Ethics*, pp. 41–42.

20. The bent-axis model was first published in: Bakken, *The Call to Wholeness*. This model was based on the foundational work of Dr. John W. Travis and Regina Sara Ryan in *Wellness Workbook* (Berkeley, CA: Ten Speed Press, 1981); expanded by Kenneth Bakken, Elaine (McCarthy) Emeth, and others in the St. Luke community.

21. Sanford, *Healing and Wholeness*, p. 33.

22. Paul Tillich, quoted in Ashley and O'Rourke, *Health Care Ethics*, p. 39.

23. Sanford, *Healing and Wholeness*, pp. 106–7.

24. Luke 9:23.

25. Harold Schulweis, "A Matter of the Heart," *Baltimore Jewish Times*, Sept. 25, 1987, p. 165. (Reprinted from *Moment* magazine.)

26. Thomas Aquinas, *Summa contra gentiles*, I.v., quoted in Matthew Fox, *Original Blessing* (Santa Fe: Bear and Company, 1983), p. 133.

27. Bakken, *The Call to Wholeness*, p. 75.

28. Ibid., p. 28.

29. Henri J. M. Nouwen, *The Genesee Diary* (Garden City, NY: Doubleday, 1976), p. 124.

30. Sanford, *Healing and Wholeness*, p. 81.

31. Stuart Kingma, quoted in Bakken, *The Call to Wholeness*, p. 29.

32. Bakken, *The Call to Wholeness*, p. 34.

CHAPTER 2: THE MEANING OF ILLNESS

1. Arthur Kleinman, MD, *The Illness Narratives* (New York: Basic Books, 1988), chap. 1.

2. Edwin H. Friedman, *Generation to Generation* (New York: The Guilford Press, 1985), pp. 14–16.

3. Leonard S. Sagan, *The Health of Nations: True Causes of Sickness and Well-Being* (New York: Basic Books, 1987), p. 202.

4. Howard Brody and David S. Sobel, "A Systems View of Health and Disease," *Ways of Health: Holistic Approaches to Ancient and Contemporary Medicine*, ed. David S. Sobel (New York: Harcourt Brace Jovanovich, 1979), p. 94.

5. Hans Selye quoted in Kenneth R. Pelletier, *Mind as Healer, Mind as Slayer* (New York: Dell, 1977), p. 3.

6. Sam Keen, "Dis-ease, Myth, and Self-Healing," workshop at Kirkridge, Bangor, PA, August 1983.

7. Jeanne Achterberg, *Imagery in Healing* (Boston: New Science Library, Shambhala, 1985), p. 84.

8. Keen, "Dis-ease, Myth, and Self-Healing" workshop.

9. John W. Travis, MD, and Regina Sara Ryan, *Wellness Workbook* (Berkeley, CA: Ten Speed Press, 1981; 2nd ed., 1988), pp. xix–xxi.

10. Keen, "Dis-ease, Myth and Self-Healing" workshop.

11. Akhter Ahsen's work described in Achterberg, *Imagery in Healing*, p. 135. For additional information read Akhter Ahsen, *Psycheye* (New York: Brandon House, 1977).

12. Luke 10:25–37.

13. Friedman, *Generation to Generation*, esp. pp. 19–39 and chap. 5.

14. Kleinman, *The Illness Narratives*, pp. 185–86.

15. Bernie S. Siegel, MD, *Love, Medicine and Miracles* (New York: Harper & Row, 1986), pp. 89–90.

16. Ibid., p. 95.

17. Achterberg, *Imagery in Healing*, chap. 4.

18. Daniel Goleman, "Study Affirms Link of Personality to Illness," *New York Times*, Jan. 19, 1988.

19. Louise L. Hay, *You Can Heal Your Life* (Santa Monica, CA: Hay House, 1984), pp. 149–88.

20. Ibid., p. 130.

21. John 9:2–3.

22. Luke 13:2–5.

23. Kleinman, *The Illness Narratives*, p. 17.

CHAPTER 3: CREATING SPACE FOR THE HOLY

1. Joseph Campbell with Bill Moyers, *The Power of Myth* (New York: Doubleday, 1988), p. 99.

2. *Living* the truth is at the heart of spiritual life. Although mind or awareness is the *gateway* to spirit, our spiritual lives are in no way dependent on our native intelligence. We *know* spirit through our mental awareness, but we do not have to be aware of spirit in order to live in harmony with it. Mentally disabled persons are able to be open to spirit, because in their unself-consciousness, they do not erect barriers to spirit.

3. M. Scott Peck, MD, *The Road Less Traveled* (New York: Touchstone, Simon and Schuster, 1978).

4. Ibid., pp. 17–18.

5. For further reading, the risks and losses of spiritual growth are explored in:.

M. Scott Peck, MD, *The Road Less Traveled* (New York: Touchstone, Simon and Schuster, 1978), and

Judith Viorst, *Necessary Losses* (New York: Simon and Schuster, 1986).

6. Evelyn Underhill, *Practical Mysticism* (Columbus, OH: Ariel Press, 1914), pp. 14–15.

7. We are indebted to Dr. James D. Whitehead and Dr. Evelyn Eaton

Whitehead for many of the concepts in this section on "Time management as spiritual discipline." The reader who is interested in further reading will find the search for the following well worth the effort:.

James D. Whitehead, "An Asceticism of Time," *Review for Religious* 39 (1980/1): 3–17; or

James D. Whitehead and Evelyn Eaton Whitehead, *Method in Ministry* (Minneapolis: Seabury, 1980), chap. 10.

8. Whitehead, "An Asceticism of Time," p. 10.

9. Gen. 32:23–33.

10. Roger Woolger, Workshop, "Touching the Spring of Vision," Common Boundary Conference, Washington, DC, Nov. 12, 1988.

11. Whitehead, "An Asceticism of Time," pp. 5–6.

12. The concept of exits within marriage is presented in Harville Hendrix' book, *Getting the Love You Want* (New York: Henry Holt and Co., 1988), pp. 92–96. We see the possibility of extending this concept to other relationships and situations, such as work, loss, and so on from which one wishes to escape.

13. Whitehead, "An Asceticism of Time," pp. 4–5, 11–15.

14. Ibid., p. 16.

15. Morton T. Kelsey, *Companions on the Inner Way* (New York: Crossroad, 1984), Ch. 6.

16. Morton Kelsey has developed a diagram that illustrates the relationship of the human person to physical and nonphysical realities, including the infinite Divine Presence, in his book, *Psychology, Medicine and Christian Healing*. We recommend this book very highly:

Morton T. Kelsey, *Psychology, Medicine and Christian Healing* (San Francisco: Harper and Row, 1988).

A diagram and explanation giving a psychological understanding of relationship between the individual and the nonphysical can be found on pp. 240–55. A diagram and explanation giving a Christian theological understanding of the same relationship can be found on pp. 279–84.

17. John A. Sanford, *Healing and Wholeness* (New York: Paulist Press, 1977), pp. 54–60.

18. Herbert Benson, MD, with Miriam Z. Klipper, *The Relaxation Response* (New York: Avon Books, 1975).

19. Richard J. Foster, *Celebration of Discipline* (San Francisco: Harper & Row, 1978), pp. 1–2.

20. 1 Kings 19:12 (KJV).

21. From the Sabbath afternoon prayer, quoted in Jacob Neusner, *The Way of the Torah* (Belmont, CA: Wadsworth Publishing Co., 1979), p. 59.

22. Sanford, *Healing and Wholeness*, p. 55.

23. Foster, *Celebration of Discipline*, p. 93.

24. Rom. 8:26–27.

25. Foster, *Celebration of Discipline*, p. 30.

26. 2 Cor. 3:17–18.

27. Hos. 2:16–17.

28. Sanford, *Healing and Wholeness*, p. 134.
29. Eph. 3:16–19.
30. Ps. 63:7–8.
31. Thich Nhat Hanh, *Being Peace* (Berkeley, CA: Parallax Press, 1987), p. 4.
32. Kenneth L. Bakken and Kathleen H. Hofeller, *The Journey Toward Wholeness* (New York: Crossroad, 1988);

Herbert Benson, MD, with Miriam Z. Klipper, *The Relaxation Response* (New York: Avon Books, 1975);

Joan Borysenko, *Minding the Body, Mending the Mind* (New York: Bantam Books, 1988);

Aryeh Kaplan, *Jewish Meditation* (New York: Schocken Books, 1985);

Stephen Levine, *A Gradual Awakening* (Garden City, NY: Anchor Press/ Doubleday, 1979);

Henri J. M. Nouwen, *With Open Hands* (Notre Dame, IN: Ave Maria Press, 1972);

M. Basil Pennington, *Centering Prayer* (Garden City, NY: Image Books, Doubleday, 1982).

Thich Nhat Hanh, *Being Peace* (Berkeley, CA: Parallax Press, 1987);
33. Morton T. Kelsey, *Adventure Inward* (Minneapolis: Augsburg, 1980), p. 34.
34. Sanford, *Healing and Wholeness*, p. 125.
35. Morton T. Kelsey, *Adventure Inward* (Minneapolis: Augsburg, 1980);

Tristine Rainer, *The New Diary* (Los Angeles: Jeremy P. Tarcher, 1978);

Louis M. Savary, Patricia H. Berne, and Strephon Kaplan Williams, *Dreams and Spiritual Growth: A Christian Approach to Dreamwork* (New York/Ramsey, NJ: Paulist Press, 1984).
36. Bernie S. Siegel, MD, *Love, Medicine and Miracles* (New York: Harper & Row, 1986), p. 97.

CHAPTER 4: A PRESCRIPTION FOR ABUNDANT LIFE

1. Evelyn Underhill, *Practical Mysticism* (Columbus, OH: Ariel Press, 1914), p. 88.
2. Ibid., p. 88.
3. Henri J. M. Nouwen, *With Open Hands* (Notre Dame, IN: Ave Maria Press, 1972), pp. 9–16.
4. Joan Borysenko, *Minding the Body, Mending the Mind* (New York: Bantam Books, 1988), p. 97–100; quote on p. 97.
5. Ibid., pp. 99–104.
6. Though neglected in the mainstream of Christianity, creation-centered spirituality is an authentic Christian tradition with historical and biblical roots and a number of highly regarded saints..

For an introduction to creation-centered spirituality, we highly recommend *Original Blessing*, by Matthew Fox. It is tempting to approach creation-centered spirituality with the same dualistic either/or thinking that it decries. We suggest holding the wisdom of *both* fall/redemption spirituality *and* creation-centered spirituality.

Matthew Fox, *Original Blessing* (Sante Fe, NM: Bear and Co., 1983).

A theological study of the Jewishness of Jesus (Yeshua) and its implications is offered in: Leonard Swidler, *Yeshua: A Model for Moderns* (Kansas City, MO: Sheed and Ward, 1988).

7. Joseph Campbell with Bill Moyers, *The Power of Myth* (New York: Doubleday, 1988), p. 107.

8. Luke 23:34.

9. John Dear, *Disarming the Heart* (New York: Paulist Press, 1987). We highly recommend this book to our readers who wish to explore nonviolence more deeply.

10. *Webster's New World Dictionary*, Third College Ed., s.v. "mercy."

11. From teaching of Thich Nhat Hanh as told in Thomas E. Clarke, S.J., "Never a Dull Moment," *Weavings* II, no. 3 (May/June 1987): 20–21.

12. Dear, *Disarming the Heart*, p. v.

13. Richard J. Foster, *Celebration of Discipline* (San Francisco: Harper & Row, 1978), p. 76.

14. Robert Bly quoted in "The Ridgeleaf," the Kirkridge newsletter, by Robert Raines, March 1989.

15. Matt. 6:21.

PART 2. TAKING CARE OF THE BODY

INTRODUCTION

1. Lawrence W. Green, Marshall W. Kreuter, Sigrid G. Deeds, and Kay B. Partridge, *Health Education Planning: A Diagnostic Approach* (Palo Alto, CA: Mayfield Publishing Co., 1980).

2. Irwin M. Rosenstock. "Adoption and Maintenance of Lifestyle Modifications," *American Journal of Preventive Medicine* 4 (1988): 349–52.

Daniel Goleman, "Breaking Bad Habits: New Therapy Focuses on the Relapse," *New York Times*, December 27, 1988, C1.

For those interested in a more detailed description see G. Alan Marlatt and Judith R. Gordon, eds., *Relapse Prevention: Maintenance Strategies in the Treatment of Addictive Behaviors* (New York: Guilford Press, 1985).

CHAPTER 5: NUTRITION AND DIET

1. US Department of Agriculture and US Department of Health and Human Services, *Dietary Guidelines for Americans*, 2d ed., 1985. Home and Garden Bulletin no. 232.

2. Department of Health and Human Services, *The Surgeon General's Report on Nutrition and Health: Summary and Recommendations*, prepared by Public Health Service, DHHS (PHS) Pub. No. 88–50211 (Washington, DC, 1988).

3. J. W. Hanson, A. P. Streissguth, and D. W. Smith, "The Effects of Moderate Alcohol Consumption During Pregnancy on Fetal Growth and Morphogenesis," *Journal of Pediatrics* 92 (1978): 457–60.

4. American Dietetic Association, "Position of the American Dietetic Association: Vegetarian Diets-Technical Support Paper," *ADA Reports 88* (March 1988): 352–54.

5. Ibid.

6. Cindy L. Wallace, Ronald Ross Watson, and Anita Ann Watson, "Reducing Cancer Risk with Vitamins C, E, and Selenium," *American Journal of Health Promotion* 3 (Summer 1988): 5–16.

7. Herman A. Tyroler, "Hypertension," in *Maxcy-Rosenau Public Health and Preventive Medicine*, 12th ed., ed. John M. Last (Norwalk, CN: Appleton-Century-Crofts, 1986), pp. 1195–1214.

8. Ibid.

9. Ron Goor and Nancy Goor, *Eater's Choice: A Food Lover's Guide to Lower Cholesterol* (Boston: Houghton Mifflin Co., 1987);

Kenneth H. Cooper, *Controlling Cholesterol* (New York: Bantam Books, 1988);

Glen C. Griffin and William P. Castelli, *Good Fat, Bad Fat: How to Lower Your Cholesterol and Beat the Odds of a Heart Attack* (Tuscon, AZ: Fisher Books, 1989);

Scott Grundy, ed., *American Heart Association Low-Fat, Low-Cholesterol Cookbook* (New York: Times Books, 1989);

Peter Kwiterovich, *Beyond Cholesterol* (Baltimore: Johns Hopkins University Press, 1989).

10. Richard S. Panush and Ella M. Webster, "Food Allergies and Other Adverse Reactions to Foods," *Medical Clinics of North America* 69 (May 1985): 533–46.

11. Department of Health and Human Services, *Health Implications of Obesity*, prepared by National Institutes of Health (Washington, DC, 1985).

12. Ibid.

13. Ibid.

14. Ibid.

15. Ibid.

16. Claude Bouchard et al, "The Response to Long-Term Overfeeding in Identical Twins," *New England Journal of Medicine* 322 (1990): 1477–82.

Albert J. Stunkard et al, "The Body-Mass Index of Twins Who Have Been Reared Apart," *New England Journal of Medicine* 322 (1990): 1483–87.

17. Candy Cummings, "Nutrition," in *Health Promotion in the Workplace*, ed. Michael P. O'Donnell and Thomas H. Ainsworth (New York: John Wiley & Sons, 1984), p. 265.

18. Ibid., p. 266.

19. John S. Spika et al., "Chloramphenicol-Resistant *Salmonella newport* Traced through Hamburger to Dairy Farms," *New England Journal of Medicine* 316 (1987): 565–70.

20. Philip Shabecoff, "100 Chemicals for Apples Add Up to Enigma on Safety," *New York Times*, February 5, 1989, 22.

21. Michael F. Jacobson, *Eater's Digest: The Consumer's Factbook of Food Additives* (New York: Anchor Books, 1976).

22. Harrison Wellford, *Sowing the Wind* (New York: Grossman Publishers, 1972). See chapter 10, "Pesticides in the Balance."

23. Richard J. Foster, *Celebration of Discipline* (New York: Harper & Row, 1978). See chapter 4, "The Discipline of Fasting."

24. Paavo Airola, *How to Keep Slim, Healthy and Young with Juice Fasting* (Phoenix: Health Plus Publishers, 1971);

Dick Gregory, *Dick Gregory's Natural Diet for Folks Who Eat* (New York: Harper & Row, 1973). See Chapter 7, "Fasting: Mother Nature's Mr. Clean";

Dori Smith, "Guidelines for a Cleansing Fast," in Berkeley Holistic Health Center, *The New Holistic Health Handbook: Living Well in a New Age,* ed. Shepherd Bliss (Lexington, MA: The Stephen Green Press, 1985), pp. 144–45.

25. Marian Burros, "What Americans Really Eat: Nutrition Can Wait," *New York Times,* January 6, 1988, C1.

26. Richard Siegel, Michael Strassfeld, and Susan Strassfeld, *The Jewish Catalog* (Philadelphia: The Jewish Publication Society of America, 1973), p. 18.

27. See Aryeh Kaplan, *Jewish Meditation: A Practical Guide* (New York: Schocken Books, 1985), especially chapter 15, "In All Your Ways," on how to make mundane acts a link to the Divine.

CHAPTER 6: HEALTH PROMOTION

1. Bob Anderson, *Stretching* (Bolinas, CA: Shelter Publications, 1980).

2. Kenneth H. Cooper, *The Aerobics Program for Total Well-Being* (New York: M. Evans and Co., 1982), and other books by Kenneth Cooper.

3. Jonathan E. Fielding, "Smoking: Health Effects and Control," *New England Journal of Medicine* 313 (1985): 491–98.

4. "Smoking in Teens Fails to Decrease Significantly," *The Nation's Health* (April 1989): 1.

5. "1986 Surgeon General's Report: The Health Consequences of Involuntary Smoking," *Morbidity and Mortality Weekly Report* 35 (December 19, 1986).

6. Jonathan E. Fielding, "Smoking and Women: Tragedy of the Majority," *New England Journal of Medicine* 317 (1987): 1343–45.

7. Department of Health and Human Services, *The Health Consequences of Smoking: Cancer,* prepared by Office on Smoking and Health (Washington, DC, 1982).

8. Charles L. Whitfield, John E. Davis, and L. Randol Barker, "Alcoholism," in *Principles of Ambulatory Medicine,* ed. L. Randol Barker et al., 2d ed. (Baltimore: Williams and Wilkins, 1986).

9. Temple Harrup and Bruce Hansen, "Substance Dependency," in *Health Promotion in the Workplace,* ed. Michael O'Donnell and Thomas Ainsworth (New York: John Wiley & Sons, 1984), pp. 447–508.

10. Whitfield et al., "Alcoholism."

11. Ibid.

12. Ibid.

13. Alan Stoudemire, Lawrence Wallack, and Nancy Hedemark, "Alcohol Dependence and Abuse," in *Closing the Gap: The Burden of Unnecessary Illness*, ed. Robert W. Amler and H. Bruce Dull (New York: Oxford University Press, 1987), pp. 9–18.

14. Paul J. Goldstein, Dana Hunt, Don C. Des Jarlais, and Sherry Deren, "Drug Dependence and Abuse," in *Closing the Gap: The Burden of Unnecessary Illness*, ed. Robert W. Amler and H. Bruce Dull (New York: Oxford University Press, 1987), pp. 89–101.

15. For an interesting discussion of this concept see Christopher Lasch, "What's Wrong with the Right," *Tikkun* 1, no. 1 (1986): 23–29.

16. James S. J. Manuso, "Management of Individual Stressors," in *Health Promotion in the Workplace*, ed. Michael P. O'Donnell and Thomas Ainsworth (New York: John Wiley & Sons, 1984), pp. 362–90.

17. Robert S. Eliot and Dennis Breo, *Is It Worth Dying For?* (New York: Bantam Books, 1984).

18. Dr. Herbert Benson, Lecture on stress and the relaxation response, Presented by The Ford Hall Forum, Broadcast by National Public Radio on November 16, 1989;

See also: Herbert Benson, MD, with Miriam Z. Klipper, *The Relaxation Response* (New York: Avon Books, 1975).

19. Robert Ornstein and David Sobel, *The Healing Brain: Breakthrough Discoveries About How the Brain Keeps Us Healthy* (New York: Touchstone, Simon and Schuster, 1988), pp. 233–39.

20. William Haddon and Susan P. Baker, "Injury Control," in *Preventive and Community Medicine*, ed. Duncan Clark and Brian MacMahon (Boston: Little, Brown & Co., 1981).

21. Ibid.

22. The National Committee for Injury Prevention and Control, *Injury Prevention: Meeting the Challenge* (New York: Oxford University Press, 1989), published as a supplement to the *American Journal of Preventive Medicine* 5, no. 3 (1989).

CHAPTER 7: DISEASE PREVENTION

1. Department of Health and Human Services, *The 1988 Report of the Joint National Committee on Detection, Evaluation, and Treatment of High Blood Pressure*, prepared by National High Blood Pressure Education Program, National Institutes of Health, NIH Pub. No. 88-1088 (Washington, DC, 1988).

2. Ibid.

3. James J. Lynch, *The Language of the Heart: The Human Body in Dialogue* (New York: Basic Books, 1985).

4. Christopher L. Melby, Roseanne M. Lyle, and Gerald C. Hyner, "Beyond Blood Pressure Screening: A Rationale for Promoting the Primary Pre-

vention of Hypertension," *American Journal of Health Promotion* 3 (Fall 1988): 5–11.

5. Department of Health and Human Services, *Report of the Expert Panel on Detection, Evaluation, and Treatment of High Blood Cholesterol in Adults (January 1988)*, prepared by National Cholesterol Education Program, National Institutes of Health, NIH Pub. No. 88-2925 (Washington, DC, 1988).

6. Craig C. White, Dennis D. Tolsma, Suzanne B. Haynes, and Daniel McGee, Jr., "Cardiovascular Disease," in *Closing the Gap: The Burden of Unnecessary Illness*, ed. Robert W. Amler and H. Bruce Dull (New York: Oxford University Press, 1987), pp. 43–54.

7. Department of Health and Human Services, *High Blood Cholesterol in Adults*.

8. Department of Health and Human Services, *Health Implications of Obesity*, prepared by National Institutes of Health (Washington, DC, 1985).

9. Ibid.

10. Meyer Friedman and Ray H. Rosenman, *Type A Behavior and Your Heart* (New York: Alfred Knopf, 1974).

11. Robert S. Eliot and Dennis Breo, *Is It Worth Dying For?* (New York: Bantam Books, 1984).

12. John C. Bailar III and Elaine M. Smith, "Progress Against Cancer?" *New England Journal of Medicine* (May 8, 1986): 1226–32.

13. Walter C. Willett and Brian MacMahon, "Diet and Cancer—An Overview," *New England Journal of Medicine* 310 (March 8, 1984): 633–38.

14. Richard Rothenberg, Philip Nasca, Mikl Jaromir, William Burnett, and Barbara Reynolds, "Cancer," in *Closing the Gap: The Burden of Unnecessary Illness*, ed. Robert W. Amler and H. Bruce Dull (New York: Oxford University Press, 1987), pp. 30–42.

15. Ibid.

16. Cindy L. Wallace, Ronald Ross Watson, and Anita Ann Watson, "Reducing Cancer Risk with Vitamins C, E, and Selenium," *American Journal of Health Promotion* 3 (Summer 1988): 5–16.

17. Ibid.

18. National Research Council, Committee on Diet, Nutrition, and Cancer, "Executive Summary: Diet, Nutrition, and Cancer," *Nutrition Today* (July/August 1982): 20–25.

19. Wallace et al., "Reducing Cancer Risk With Vitamins C, E, and Selenium."

20. Ibid.

21. Walter C. Willett and Brian MacMahon, "Diet and Cancer—An Overview," *New England Journal of Medicine* 310 (March 15, 1984): 697–703.

22. Walter Willett and Brian MacMahon, "Diet and Cancer," *New England Journal of Medicine* 310 (March 8, 1984): 633–38.

23. Willett and MacMahon, "Diet and Cancer," *New England Journal of Medicine* 310 (March 15, 1984): 697–703.

24. Department of Health and Human Services, *Diet, Nutrition, and Cancer*

Prevention: The Good News, prepared by National Cancer Institute, National Institutes of Health, NIH Pub. No. 87-2878 (Washington, DC, 1986).

25. Ibid.

26. "Can Eating the 'Right' Food Cut Your Risk of Cancer?" *Tufts University Diet & Nutrition Letter* 6 (April 1988): 3–6.

27. Rothenberg et al., "Cancer."

28. R. Doll and R. Peto, *The Causes of Cancer: Quantitative Estimates of Avoidable Risks of Cancer in the United States Today* (New York: Oxford University Press, 1981).

29. R. L. Stern et al., *Archives of Dermatology* 122 (1986): 537; quoted in "Sunscreens," *The Medical Letter* 30 (June 17, 1988): 62.

30. David B. Thomas, "Cancer," in *Public Health and Preventive Medicine,* 12th ed., ed. John Last (Norwalk, CN: Appleton) Century–Crofts, 1986), pp. 1133–58.

31. US Preventive Services Task Force, "Screening for Lung Cancer," chap. 10 in *Guide to Clinical Preventive Services* (Washington, DC, 1989).

32. Rothenberg et al., "Cancer."

33. Sandra Blakeslee, "New Tests Can Detect Viruses That Signal Risk of Cervical Cancer," *New York Times,* October 20, 1988, B15.

34. US Preventive Services Task Force, "Screening for Cervical Cancer," chap. 8 in *Guide to Clinical Preventive Services* (Washington, DC, 1989).

35. Rothenberg et al., "Cancer."

36. Ibid.

37. US Preventive Services Task Force, "Screening for Breast Cancer," chap. 6 in *Guide to Clinical Preventive Services* (Washington, DC, 1989).

38. Ibid.

39. Kenneth C. Chu, Charles R. Smart, and Robert E. Tarone, "Analysis of Breast Cancer Mortality and Stage Distribution by Age for the Health Insurance Plan Clinical Trial," *Journal of the National Cancer Institute* 80 (September 21, 1988): 1125–32.

40. US Preventive Services Task Force, "Screening for Colorectal Cancer," chap. 7 in *Guide to Clinical Preventive Services* (Washington, DC, 1989).

41. Ibid.

42. Department of Health and Human Services, *Surgeon General's Report on Acquired Immune Deficiency Syndrome,* prepared by Public Health Service (Washington, DC, 1986).

43. Centers for Disease Control, "Human Immunodeficiency Virus Infection in the United States: A Review of Current Knowledge," *Morbidity and Mortality Weekly Report* 36 (1987): supplement no. S–6.

44. Richard N. L. Andrews and Alvis G. Turner, "Controlling Toxic Chemicals in the Environment," in *Toxic Chemicals, Health, and the Environment,* ed. Lester B. Lave and Arthur C. Upton (Baltimore: Johns Hopkins University Press, 1987), pp. 5–37.

45. G. B. Gerber, A. Leonard, and P. Jacquet, "Toxicity, Mutagenicity, and Teratogenicity of Lead," *Mutation Research* 76 (1980): 115–41.

46. Marvin S. Legator, Barbara L. Harper, and Michael J. Scott, eds., *The Health Detective's Handbook: A Guide to the Investigation of Environmental Health Hazards by Nonprofessionals* (Baltimore: Johns Hopkins University Press, 1985).

47. Andrews and Turner, "Controlling Toxic Chemicals in the Environment."

CHAPTER 8: HEALTHY RELATIONSHIPS

1. John A. Sanford, *Healing and Wholeness* (New York: Paulist Press, 1977), p. 120.

2. This composite list is based on the foundational work of Delores Curran and Charles Whitfield, plus our own ideas:

Delores Curran, *Traits of a Healthy Family* (New York: Ballantine, 1983);

Charles L. Whitfield, MD, *Healing the Child Within* (Pompano Beach, FL: Health Communications, 1987), p. 18.

3. Whitfield, *Healing the Child Within*, p. 2.

4. Anne Wilson Schaef, *When Society Becomes an Addict* (San Francisco: Harper & Row, 1987), p. 29.

5. Gerald G. May, MD, *Addiction and Grace* (San Francisco: Harper & Row, 1988), p. 24. Highly recommended reading!

6. Recommended reading:.

Anne Wilson Schaef, *When Society Becomes an Addict* (San Francisco: Harper & Row, 1987); and

Anne Wilson Schaef and Diane Fassel, *The Addictive Organization* (San Francisco: Harper & Row, 1988).

7. May, *Addiction and Grace*, quote from p. 11.

8. Ibid.

9. Schaef, *When Society Becomes an Addict*, p. 25.

10. This chart is a composite based on foundational work of Melody Beattie, John Bradshaw, Gerald May, Pia Mellody, and Charles Whitfield.

11. Harville Hendrix, PhD, *Getting the Love You Want* (New York: Henry Holt and Co., 1988).

12. Pia Mellody, with Andrea Wells Miller and J. Keith Miller, *Facing Codependence* (San Francisco: Harper & Row, 1989), esp. chap. 4.

13. Nathaniel Branden, *The Psychology of Romantic Love* (New York: Bantam Books, 1981), pp. 140–60.

14. The compilations of traits of a healthy marriage and traits of a healthy family are based in part on the work of Delores Curran and James L. Framo, PhD:

Delores Curran, *Traits of a Healthy Family* (New York: Ballantine Books, 1983);

James L. Framo, PhD, "The Integration of Marital Therapy with Sessions with Family of Origin," in *Handbook of Family Therapy*, ed. Alan S. Gurman, PhD, and David P. Kniskern, PsyD (New York: Brunner/Mazel, 1981), pp. 139–40.

15. Melody Beattie, *Codependent No More* (New York: Harper/Hazeldon, 1987).

Dr. Susan Forward with Craig Buck, *Toxic Parents* (New York: Bantam Books, 1989);

Herbert L. Gravitz and Julie D. Bowden, *Recovery: A Guide for Adult Children of Alcoholics* (New York: Simon & Schuster, 1985);

Harville Hendrix, PhD, *Getting the Love You Want* (New York: Henry Holt & Co., 1988);

Harriet Goldhor Lerner, PhD, *The Dance of Anger* (New York: Harper & Row, 1985);

Harriet Goldhor Lerner, PhD, *The Dance of Intimacy* (New York: Harper & Row, 1989);

Pia Mellody, with Andrea Wells Miller and J. Keith Miller, *Facing Codependence* (San Francisco: Harper & Row, 1989);

Charles L. Whitfield, MD, *Healing the Child Within* (Pompano Beach, FL: Health Communications, 1987).

16. Matt. 7:1–5; Luke 6:41–42.

17. Edwin H. Friedman, *Generation to Generation* (New York: Guilford Press, 1985), pp. 132–34.

18. Stephanie Matthews Simonton, *The Healing Family* (New York: Bantam Books, 1984), pp. 16–20;

Bernie S. Siegel, MD, *Love, Medicine and Miracles* (New York: Harper & Row, 1986), pp. 92–96.

19. Arthur Kleinman, MD, *The Illness Narratives* (New York: Basic Books, 1988), p. 181.

20. Henri Nouwen, "The Peace That Is Not of this World," *Weavings* III (March/April 1988) : pp. 23–34.

Jean Vanier, "The Secret of the Gospel," *The Other Side* (March, 1986), pp. 18–23.

21. Gen. 32:23–32.

CHAPTER 9: HEALING PRESENCE

1. *Webster's New World Dictionary*, 3d College Ed., s.v. "compassion."

2. Henri J. M. Nouwen, *The Wounded Healer* (Garden City, NY: Image Books, 1979), p. 72.

3. Stephen Levine, *Healing into Life and Death* (Garden City, NY: Anchor Press/Doubleday, 1987), pp. 66–76.

4. Nouwen, *The Wounded Healer*, p. 91.

5. Morton T. Kelsey, *Caring* (New York: Paulist Press, 1981), p. 68.

6. Based on M. Scott Peck, MD, *The Road Less Traveled* (New York: Touchstone, Simon and Schuster, 1978), p. 81.

7. Sherry Suib Cohen, *The Magic of Touch*, (New York: Harper & Row, 1987).

8. Research of James W. Prescott, "Body Pleasure and the Origins of Violence," *The Futurist*, vol. 9, no. 2 (1975): 64–74.

Cited in James B. Nelson, *The Intimate Connection* (Philadelphia: The Westminster Press, 1988), p. 80.

9. Bernie S. Siegel, MD, *Love, Medicine and Miracles* (New York: Harper & Row, 1986), especially chaps. 2 and 3.

10. Akhter Ahsen, *Psycheye* (New York: Brandon House, 1977).

11. In cases of overwhelming trauma, the memory may split: the emotional and physical somatic content, the mental picture, and the interpretation are stored separately in the unconscious. The different components of the memory may surface in spontaneous altered states, such as flashbacks. For example, it is not unusual for adult survivors of childhood sexual abuse to have emotional flashbacks without a mental picture, or mental pictures of events from the past without emotion. (An understanding of the split-off, encapsulated wound of sexual abuse survivors has been developed by Dr. Gary M. Lee.) This phenomena causes many to doubt the truth of the memory fragment; however, these fragmented eidetics are just as real as those that are intact.

12. Ernest Lawrence Rossi, *The Psychobiology of Mind-Body Healing*, (New York: W. W. Norton and Co., 1986), pp. 36–40.

13. Ibid., chap. 5.

14. Jeanne Achterberg, *Imagery in Healing* (Boston: New Science Library, Shambhala, 1985), pp. 122–24.

15. Rossi, *The Psychobiology of Mind-Body Healing*, p. 19.

16. Jeanne Achterberg, *Imagery in Healing* (Boston: New Science Library, Shambhala, 1985);

Steven Locke, MD, and Douglas Colligan, *The Healer Within* (New York: New American Library, 1986);

Ernest Lawrence Rossi, *The Psychobiology of Mind-Body Healing* (New York: W. W. Norton and Co., 1986).

17. Bernie S. Siegel, MD, *Love, Medicine and Miracles* (New York: Harper & Row, 1986);

Bernie S. Siegel, MD, *Peace, Love and Healing* (New York: Harper & Row, 1989);

Gregg M. Furth, *The Secret World of Drawings* (Boston: Sigo Press, 1988).

18. O. Carl Simonton, MD, Stephanie Matthews-Simonton, and James L. Creighton, *Getting Well Again* (New York: Bantam Books, 1980), chaps. 11 & 12.

19. Mark 11:24.

20. Matt. 17:20; Luke 17:6.

21. Gerald G. May, MD, *Addiction and Grace* (San Francisco: Harper & Row, 1988), p. 128.

22. Herbert Benson, MD, with William Proctor, *Beyond the Relaxation Response* (New York: Times Books, 1984), quote p. 8.

23. 2 Cor. 4:7.

Recommended Reading

HEALING AND WHOLENESS

Achterberg, Jeanne. *Imagery in Healing*. Boston: New Science Library, Shambhala, 1985.

Bakken, Kenneth L. *The Call to Wholeness*. New York: Crossroad, 1986.

—— and Hofeller, Kathleen H. *The Journey Toward Wholeness*. New York: Crossroad, 1988.

Brewi, Janice, and Brennan, Anne. *Celebrate Mid-Life*. New York: Crossroad, 1988.

Kelsey, Morton T. *Psychology, Medicine and Christian Healing*. San Francisco: Harper & Row, 1988.

Kleinman, Arthur, MD. *The Illness Narratives*. New York: Basic Books, 1988.

Levine, Stephen. *Healing into Life and Death*. Garden City, NY: Anchor Press/Doubleday, 1987.

Locke, Steven, MD, and Colligan, Douglas. *The Healer Within*. New York: New American Library, 1986.

May, Gerald G., MD. *Addiction and Grace*. San Francisco: Harper and Row, 1988.

Peck, M. Scott, MD. *The Road Less Traveled*. New York: Touchstone, Simon and Schuster, 1978.

Sanford, John A. *Healing and Wholeness*. New York: Paulist Press, 1977.

Siegel, Bernie S., MD. *Love, Medicine and Miracles*. New York: Harper & Row, 1986.

Travis, John W., MD, and Ryan, Regina Sara. *Wellness Workbook* (2d ed.). Berkeley, CA: Ten Speed Press, 1988.

FAMILY AND RELATIONSHIPS

Beattie, Melody. *Codependent No More*. New York: Harper/Hazelden, 1987.

Berends, Polly Berrien. *Whole Child / Whole Parent*. New York: Harper & Row, 1987.

Bradshaw, John. *Bradshaw On: The Family*. Pompano Beach, FL: Health Communications, 1988.

Curran, Delores. *Traits of a Healthy Family*. New York: Ballantine, 1983.

Forward, Susan, PhD, with Buck, Craig. *Toxic Parents*. New York: Bantam Books, 1989.

Friedman, Edwin H. *Generation to Generation*. New York: Guilford Press, 1985.

Gravitz, Herbert L., and Bowden, Julie D. *Recovery: A Guide for Adult Children of Alcoholics*. New York: Simon and Schuster, 1985.

Hendrix, Harville, PhD. *Getting the Love You Want*. New York: Henry Holt and Co., 1988.

Lerner, Harriet Goldhor, PhD. *The Dance of Anger*. New York: Harper & Row, 1985.

―――― *The Dance of Intimacy*. New York: Harper & Row, 1989.

Mellody, Pia, with Miller, Andrea Wells, and Miller, J. Keith. *Facing Codependence*. San Francisco: Harper & Row, 1989.

Schaef, Anne Wilson. *When Society Becomes an Addict*. San Francisco: Harper & Row, 1987.

Simonton, Stephanie Matthews. *The Healing Family*. New York: Bantam Books, 1984.

Whitfield, Charles L. *Healing the Child Within*. Pompano Beach, FL: Health Communications, 1987.

TOOLS FOR WELLBEING

Anderson, Bob. *Stretching*. Bolinas, CA: Shelter Publications, 1980.

Belsky, Janet K. *Here Tomorrow: Making the Most of Life after Fifty*. Baltimore: Johns Hopkins University Press, 1988.

Benson, Herbert, MD, with Klipper, Miriam Z. *The Relaxation Response*. New York: Avon Books, 1975.

―――― with Proctor, William. *Beyond the Relaxation Response*. New York: Times Books, 1984.

Borysenko, Joan. *Minding the Body, Mending the Mind*. New York: Bantam Books, 1988.

Brody, Jane E. *Jane Brody's Nutrition Book: A Lifetime Guide to Good Eating for Better Health and Weight Control*. New York: Bantam Books, 1987.

Cooper, Kenneth H. *The Aerobics Program for Total Well-Being*. New York: Bantam Books, 1982.

Dreher, Henry. *Your Defense Against Cancer: The Complete Guide to Prevention*. New York: Harper & Row, 1988.

Edwards, Tilden. *Spiritual Friend*. New York: Paulist Press, 1980.

Foster, Richard J. *Celebration of Discipline*. New York: Harper & Row, 1978.

Goor, Ron and Goor, Nancy. *Eater's Choice: A Food Lover's Guide to Lower Cholesterol*. Boston: Houghton Mifflin Co., 1987.

Hart, Thomas N. *The Art of Christian Listening*. New York: Paulist Press, 1980.

Kaplan, Aryeh. *Jewish Meditation: A Practical Guide*. New York: Schocken Books, 1985.

Kelsey, Morton T. *Adventure Inward*. Minneapolis: Augsburg, 1980.

―――― *Caring*. New York: Paulist Press, 1981.

Legator, Marvin S., Harper, Barbara L., and Scott, Michael J. (eds.). *The Health Detective's Handbook: A Guide to the Investigation of Environmental Health Hazards by Nonprofessionals*. Baltimore: Johns Hopkins University Press, 1985.

Levine, Stephen. *A Gradual Awakening*. Garden City, NY: Anchor Press/ Doubleday, 1979.

Lingle, Virginia A. and Wood, M. Sandra. *How to Find Information About AIDS*. New York: Harrington Park Press, 1988.

The National Committee for Injury Prevention and Control. *Injury Prevention: Meeting the Challenge*. New York: Oxford University Press, 1989 (supplement to *American Journal of Preventive Medicine 5*, No. 3, 1989).

Nouwen, Henri J. M. *With Open Hands*. Notre Dame, IN: Ave Maria Press, 1972.

Pennington, M. Basil, OCSO. *Centering Prayer*. Garden City, NY: Image Books, Doubleday, 1982.

Rainer, Tristine. *The New Diary*. Los Angeles: Jeremy P. Tarcher, 1978.

Savary, Louis M., Berne, Patricia H., and Williams, Strephon Kaplan. *Dreams and Spiritual Growth*. New York: Paulist Press, 1984.

Simonton, O. Carl, MD; Matthews-Simonton, Stephanie; and Creighton, James L. *Getting Well Again*. New York: Bantam Books, 1980.

Thich Nhat Hanh. *Being Peace*. Berkeley, CA: Parallax Press, 1987.

Whitehead, James D. "An Asceticism of Time" *Review for Religious* 39 (1980/ 1): 3-17; or

—— and Whitehead, Evelyn Eaton. *Method in Ministry*. Minneapolis: Seabury, 1980, chap. 10.

Index